Simplified Interpretation of Pacemaker ECGs

Aaron B. Hesselson, MD, BSE, FACC
Assistant Clinical Professor of Medicine
Wayne State University School of Medicine
Detroit, Michigan

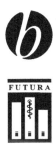

Futura, an imprint of Blackwell Publishing

Blackwell Publishing, Inc./Futura Division, 3 West Main Street, Elmsford, New York 10523, USA

Blackwell Publishing, Inc., 350 Main Street, Malden, Massachusetts 02148-5018, USA

Blackwell Publishing Ltd, 9600 Garsington Road, Oxford OX4 2DQ, UK

Blackwell Science Asia Pty Ltd, 550 Swanston Street, Carlton South, Victoria 3053, Australia

02 03 04 05 5 4 3 2 1

10   2010

Library of Congress Cataloging-in-Publication Data
Hesselson, Aaron B.
    Simplified interpretation of pacemaker ECGs / Aaron B. Hesselson.
        p. ; cm.
    Includes index.
    ISBN 978-1-4051-0372-5 (alk. paper)
    1. Cardiac pacing.   2. Electrocardiography,   I. Title.
    [DNLM: 1. Electrocardiography–methods–Case Report. 2. Cardiac
Pacing, Artificial–Case Report. 3. Electrocardiography–instrumentation–Case
Report. 4. Pacemaker, Artificial–Case Report. WG 140 H587s 2003]
    RC684.P3H47 2003
    617.4'120645–dc21   2003004824

A catalogue record for this title is available from the British Library

For further information on Blackwell Publishing, visit our website:
www.futuraco.com
www.blackwellpublishing.com

Notice: The indications and dosages of all drugs in this book have been recommended in the medical literature and conform to the practices of the general community. The medications described do not necessarily have specific approval by the Food and Drug Administration for use in the diseases and dosages for which they are recommended. The package insert for each drug should be consulted for use and dosage as approved by the FDA. Because standards for usage change, it is advisable to keep abreast of revised recommendations, particularly those concerning new drugs.

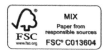

For Heather

Foreword

Within the past three decades, pacemakers have evolved from fixed-rate, single-chamber units to incredibly sophisticated dual-chamber devices that are capable of many different pacing modalities, that provide physiologic response to exercise or stress using a variety of sensors, and that also provide various diagnostic capabilities. These advances in technology have been accompanied by an inevitable increase in the complexity of ECG interpretation of pacemaker-generated rhythms. For those not directly involved in the management of pacemakers, the attainment of the skills needed to interpret pacemaker ECGs has been a daunting task.

With the availability of *Simplified Interpretation of Pacemaker ECGs*, a previously daunting task is now simple and painless. The reader is led step-by-step through all of the information needed to interpret pacemaker ECGs. After a brief refresher course on basic ECG interpretation, the reader is provided with an overview of the conduction system of the heart. The hardware associated with pacing is then reviewed, followed by an explanation of sensing and pacing function of pacemakers. Next is an explanation of the most common pacing modalities in a fashion that is simple to understand, yet thorough enough to make pacemaker ECG interpretation easy. This is followed by a very useful section dealing with miscellaneous topics such as automatic threshold determination, electromagnetic interference, and the use of pacing for indications other than bradycardia. The text ends with a series of case studies that brings together all of the information learned and provides the reader with a self-assessment of the topics that may need additional review.

The text is replete with schematic illustrations, charts, and ECG recordings that greatly enhance the learning experience. Furthermore, the reader is frequently challenged to answer questions that reinforce the material learned in a particular section.

Dr. Hesselson has succeeded admirably in distilling a potentially confusing body of knowledge into a simple-to-understand and palatable programmed text that is fun to go through. He could have entitled the book *Pacemakers for Dummies*. With the few hours of time needed to go through this book, no one need feel like a "dummy" when faced with a pacemaker ECG.

Fred Morady, MD
Professor of Medicine
Director, Clinical Electrophysiology Laboratory
University of Michigan Medical Center
Ann Arbor, MI

Preface

It was 12 years ago that I began working in my first job out of college as a clinical pacemaker research engineer at Beth Israel Medical Center in Newark, NJ. Not having much experience with ECG interpretation I was given a basic text to read and learn. Soon after that I was ready to begin learning pacemaker ECG interpretation, and was surprised to find out that a similar basic text solely dedicated to pacemaker ECGs did not exist. Instead I was given technical manuals, proprietary "learning manuals" from various pacemaker manufacturers, and a pacemaker with a heart rhythm simulator to work with. For an engineer these were not difficult to use and understand.

Having since gone to medical school and trained as an internist, cardiologist, and now cardiac electrophysiologist, I have found that this lack of a basic pacemaker ECG interpretation text still exists. This book intends to change that. It has been written with a few thoughts in mind: "what would I have wanted in my hands when I was just beginning to learn pacemaker ECGs?" and "keep it as simple as possible so that not only an engineer, but also nurses, technicians, and even physicians can follow." I have attempted to concentrate on the ideas that I found best in my experience. As such, there is an enormous emphasis placed on knowing a few basic parameters of the pacemaker system and their relation to the patient's native heart rate and integrity of conduction from atrium to ventricle. The book requires that one already have a working knowledge of basic non-pacemaker ECG interpretation. Once studied, even fairly difficult pacemaker ECGs should be appropriately interpreted.

As one will see when reading the text, the figures are not numbered. Each image is placed in direct proximity to the text that refers to it. Also, there are fill-in-the-blank questions, with answers in boldface directly below, following most paragraphs. This "programmed teaching" style is done to emphasize salient points in the preceding text. In order to help maintain this format, there may be empty areas on some pages. One may optimally use these spaces for study notes.

Some pacemakers have functions that are peculiar to the individual model and that may affect the ECG. Such details are not emphasized here. Consulting the technical manual that comes with each pacemaker, the local pacemaker ECG guru (EP attending, nurse, whoever), or pacemaker manufacturer technical service/sales representative is helpful in this regard. Good luck!

Acknowledgments

The following were instrumental influences, without whom this book would not be possible: Victor Parsonnet, MD; Alan D. Bernstein, EngScD; Donna Neglia, RN; Esther Schilling, RN; Ralph Gallagher; Thomas M. Bashore, MD, Robert Sorrentino, MD; Ruth Ann Greenfield, MD; and Matthew Flemming, MD.

Contents

Section III
Unusual Pacing Situations and Alternate Applications of Permanent Pacing

Section IV
Case Studies

Section I

The Basics

Chapter 1

Basic ECG Refresher

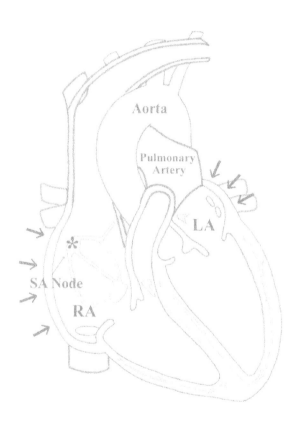

It is strongly suggested that one master basic non-pacemaker electrocardiograph (ECG) interpretation before beginning pacemaker ECG analysis. What follows in this section is not meant to provide that skill. Rather this "refresher" is meant to highlight some areas of ECG interpretation that may be pertinent to understanding pacemaker rhythms and device function. Those who already feel comfortable in their non-pacemaker ECG interpretative skills should proceed beyond this section.

ECG "ANATOMY"

The sinus or "SA node" is the heart's own pacemaker that, in normal circumstances, initiates the heartbeat. From this native activation first the right (RA) and then left atrium (LA) are stimulated to contract. This activation is noted on the ECG as a "P wave."

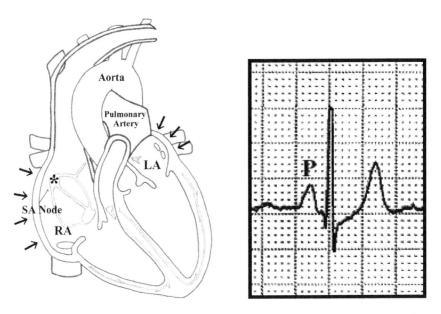

Atrial electrical activation is represented on the ECG by the ———.

The structure in the RA that normally initiates the heartbeat is the ———.

P WAVE
SA or SINUS NODE

After atrial activation, the "atrioventricular (AV) node," followed by the "His bundle," and then the "left (LBB)" and "right (RBB) bundle branches" become electrically stimulated. This results in left (LV) and right (RV) ventricular contraction, and is noted on the ECG as a "QRS" complex.* The ventricles then relax after contraction. This event, "ventricular repolarization," is noted on the ECG as the "T wave."

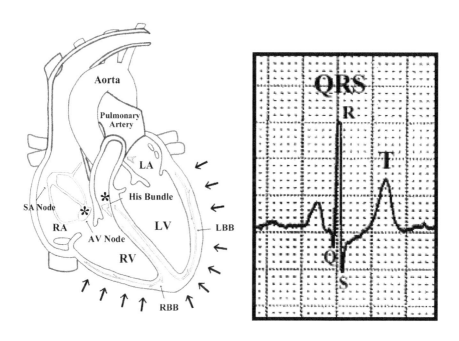

The QRS complex on an ECG represents _____ electrical activation.

Ventricular _____ is seen on the ECG as the T wave.

VENTRICULAR REPOLARIZATION

*QRS is a generic term that refers to the ventricular complex on the surface ECG. Not every QRS complex has all three components: Q wave (the initial negative deflection), R wave (the initial positive deflection), and S wave (negative deflection after an R wave). In some cases there is a second positive component termed R′.

HOW FAST IS IT?

An easy method for determining how fast the heart rate is, on a standard speed ECG grid, is to find a QRS complex on a heavy grid line and note where the next QRS falls. The subsequent heavy grid lines after the first correspond to heart rates of 300, 150, 100, 75, 60, and 50 beats per minute (bpm), respectively. By memorizing this grid line progression, quickly approximating heart rate becomes simple!

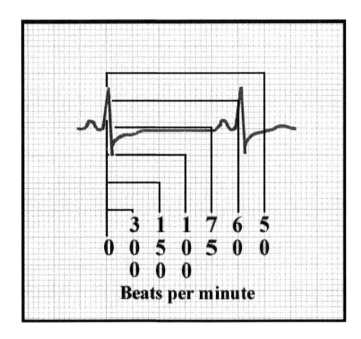

The heart rate when a second QRS complex occurs four heavy grid lines after the first is _____.

A heart rate of 150 bpm would occur when two QRS complexes occur _____ heavy grid lines apart.

75 bpm
2

Selected Arrhythmias

Normally the sinus node causes the heart to beat anywhere between 60 and 100 bpm at rest. When the sinus rate is less than 60 bpm the rhythm is termed "sinus bradycardia."

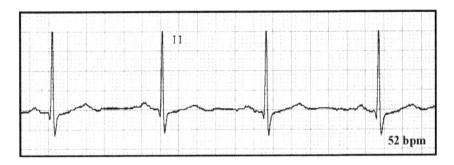

When the sinus rate is greater than 100 bpm the rhythm is termed "sinus tachycardia."

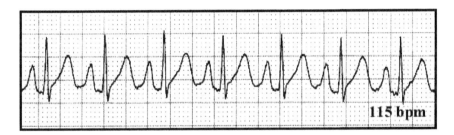

Sinus rhythms that are less than 60 bpm and greater than 100 bpm are, respectively, called sinus _____ and _____.

BRADYCARDIA, TACHYCARDIA

It can rarely happen that neither the sinus node nor any other site in the atria initiate a heartbeat. In this instance the ventricles may respond, on their own, with what is called a "junctional" heart rhythm. The rate is typically less than 60 bpm and can frequently require pacemaker treatment!

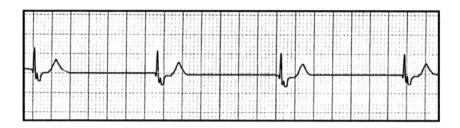

Even rarer is the occurrence of a complete lack of heart rhythm or "asystole." Asystole may occur in the setting of significant cardiac abnormalities and frequently demands a pacemaker to help maintain a heart rhythm.

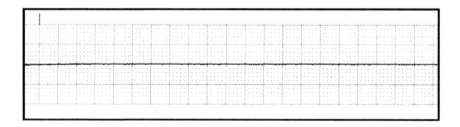

A junctional rhythm may result when no _____ site initiates a heartbeat.

_____ is the term used to define a complete lack of a heart rhythm.

ATRIAL
ASYSTOLE

The most common abnormal heart rhythm is "atrial fibrillation" (AF). It occurs when numerous sites in the atria other than the sinus node fire at the same time to make the atria beat. A rapid chaotic atrial rhythm that has an irregularly irregular characteristic to its conducted ventricular rate is the usual result. Instead of P waves, "fibrillation waves" may frequently be seen on the ECG.

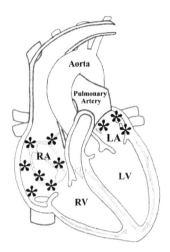

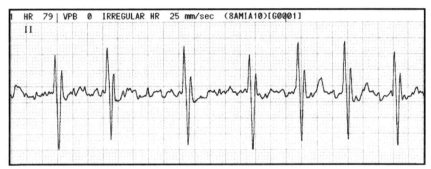

It is not unusual to have a pause and/or a bradycardic rhythm result if AF suddenly ceases, especially in elderly patients.

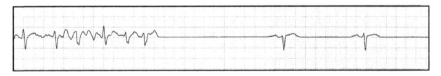

This situation is part of a sinus node abnormality called "sick sinus syndrome" and can frequently require a pacemaker to treat.

AF is classically characterized by an _____ _____ ventricular response.

There are no __ _____ in AF.

IRREGULARLY IRREGULAR
P WAVES

A "cousin" of AF is atrial flutter. With this rhythm the atria again beat rapidly but in an organized fashion between 240 and 300 bpm. Again no P waves are seen but classic "saw-tooth" flutter waves are frequently discernible on the ECG in a typical variety. Typical atrial flutter comes from a single reentrant electric circuit (like a dog chasing its tail) in the RA.

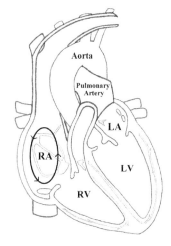

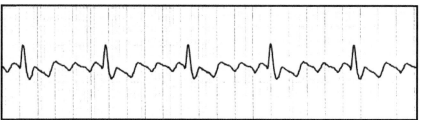

Both AF and atrial flutter may make the ventricles beat very rapidly depending on how fast the AV node allows signals to be transported to them.

Typical atrial flutter is characterized by ＿＿＿＿ ＿＿＿＿ flutter waves on the ECG.

The atria beat in an ＿＿＿＿ fashion in atrial flutter.

AF and atrial flutter may both make the ventricles beat very ＿＿＿＿.

SAW TOOTH
ORGANIZED
RAPIDLY

In certain circumstances the ventricles may beat very rapidly on their own from a single source in either the LV or RV. The ventricular rhythm may be organized and occur at rates from 110 to 250 bpm. This is called "ventricular tachycardia" (VT).

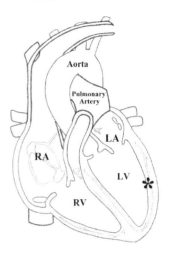

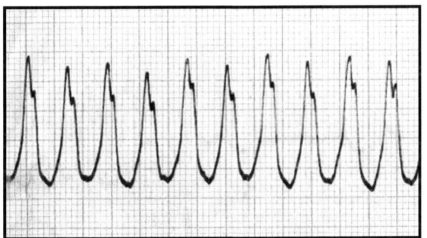

VT may cause significant symptoms and can be deadly if it is sustained!

The rate of VT is generally _____ to _____ bpm.

If it is sustained _____ can cause significant symptoms or even death!

110, 250
VT

Another rapid ventricular rhythm, this one completely chaotic (i.e., akin to AF but in the ventricles), is "ventricular fibrillation." This rhythm renders the heart ineffective in producing any organized pumping action and *is* deadly if it is sustained and not treated!

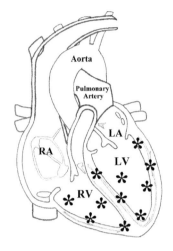

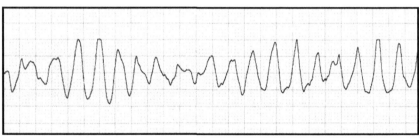

VF produces no _____ pumping action and is _____ if sustained and not treated!

ORGANIZED, DEADLY

The "Blocks"

The interval from the beginning of the P wave to the onset of the QRS complex is called the "PR interval." It is an important measurement because prolongation of the interval is indicative of a delay, or "block," in electrical conduction at some point between the atria and the ventricles.

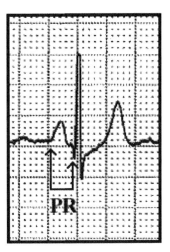

"First-degree" AV block occurs when there is a fixed prolongation of the PR interval greater than 200 ms (>1 big ECG grid box).

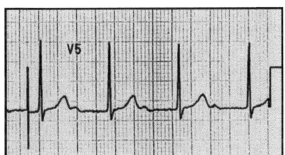

With first-degree AV block there is a ventricular beat for every atrial beat, or in other words, each atrial beat conducts down to the ventricles.

The PR interval is measured from the beginning of the ___ _____ to the onset of the _____ complex.

The PR interval is greater than _____ ____ and is _____ in first-degree AV block.

Each atrial beat _____ conduct to the ventricles in first-degree AV block.

P WAVE, QRS
200 ms, FIXED
DOES

"Second-degree AV block" occurs when sinus beats intermittently do not conduct to the ventricles. It comes in two basic varieties, "Mobitz type I" and "Mobitz type II."

There is a gradual prolongation of the PR interval with each successive beat before conduction block to the ventricles occurs with second-degree AV block Mobitz type I.

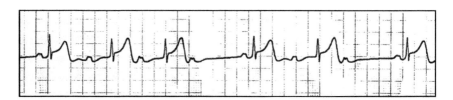

The PR interval remains fixed in second-degree AV block Mobitz type II before conduction does not occur. This may result in single or multiple nonconducted beats, as in below.

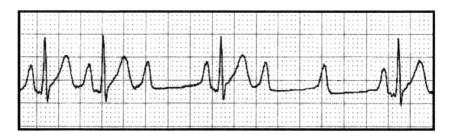

With second-degree AV block P waves are _____ not conducted to the ventricle.

The PR interval is fixed in Mobitz type ____ and progressively lengthens in Mobitz type ____ second-degree AV block before conduction block occurs.

INTERMITTENTLY
II, I

"Third-degree AV block" or "complete heart block" occurs when no atrial beats conduct to the ventricles. The atrial and ventricular rhythms bear no relationship to each other. The ventricular rhythm is slower (typically ≤50 bpm) or even completely absent!

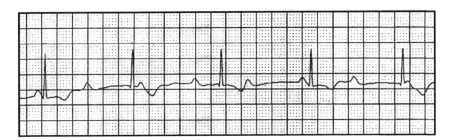

Both second- and third-degree AV block may require a pacemaker to be implanted depending on the cause of the block and the patient's symptoms!

_____ atrial beats conduct to the ventricles in complete heart block and can frequently require a _____ to treat.

In complete heart block the atrial and ventricular rhythms bear no _____ to each other.

With complete heart block the ventricular rhythm may be _____ or even completely _____.

NO, PACEMAKER
RELATIONSHIP
SLOW, ABSENT

Another form of conduction block is suggested when the width of the QRS complex is prolonged. If the QRS complex width is greater than 3 small grid boxes on the ECG, then a block in electrical conduction in one of the bundle branches may likely have occurred. The bundle branch that is blocked can be determined by analyzing the morphology of the QRS complex on the surface 12-lead ECG, particularly in chest leads V_1 and/or V_6.

Right bundle branch block (RBBB) is noted particularly in chest lead V_1 as a wide QRS complex with, most commonly, an R-S-R' morphology.

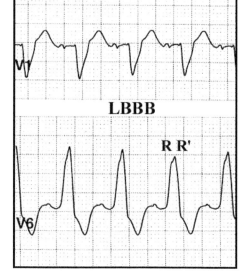

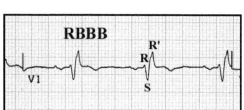

Left bundle branch block (LBBB) appears commonly as a wide QRS complex with a slight R-R' notching in its peak in chest lead V_6. Note how different RBBB and LBBB appear. This difference will become important for determining appropriate function in ventricular pacing systems.

Bundle branch block in and of itself is not typically an indication for a pacemaker to be implanted.

Characteristically, LBBB has an _____ morphology in chest lead _____, while RBBB has an _____ morphology in chest lead _____.

R-R', V_6, R-S-R', V_1

PREMATURE ATRIAL COMPLEXES AND PREMATURE VENTRICULAR COMPLEXES

Premature beats may occur when a single ectopic source spontaneously discharges from anywhere in either the atrium or ventricle. In the case of a premature atrial complex (PAC) the P wave morphology usually appears different from that of sinus rhythm and occurs earlier than expected.

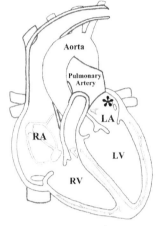

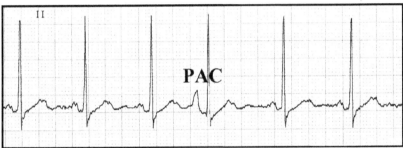

If a PAC occurs early enough it may not conduct to the ventricles. This is a normal occurrence and does not necessarily indicate a form of second-degree AV block.

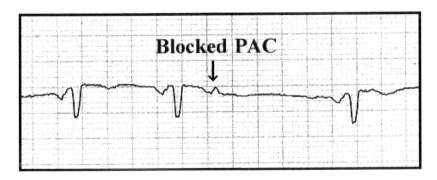

A _____ may originate anywhere in the atria and give rise to a P wave that has a _____ morphology than that of a sinus rhythm P wave.

PACs occurring significantly early may not _____ to the ventricles.

PAC, DIFFERENT CONDUCT

Similarly, a premature ventricular complex (PVC) typically appears greatly different than the QRS complex from normal conduction and also occurs earlier than the next expected beat. The difference in appearance is because the ectopic site causes one ventricle of the heart to be activated before the other, giving the appearance of bundle branch block. The bundle branch block likeness depends on whether the PVC originates in the LV (RBBB appearance) versus the RV (LBBB appearance). Continuous firing of the ventricular ectopic site can give rise to VT!

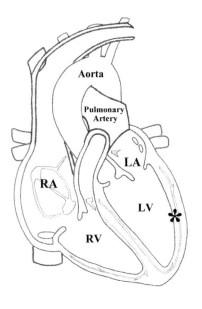

A PVC may also cause conduction to occur backward to the atrium. This is called "retrograde conduction" and gives rise to a "retrograde P wave."

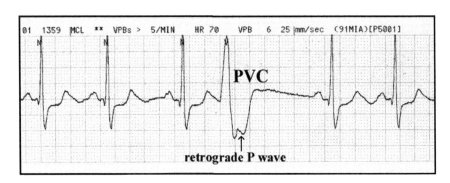

A PVC originating in the RV tends to appear with an _____ morphology.

A _____ P wave occurs when conduction proceeds _____ from the ventricles to the atria.

LBBB
RETROGRADE, BACKWARD

Chapter 2

What Is a Pacemaker?

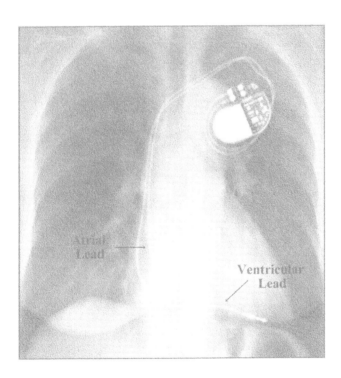

Atrial
Lead

Ventricular
Lead

WHAT IS A PACEMAKER?

In patients whose heart rates have a tendency to become too slow a physician may prescribe and implant a specialized electronic device called a pacemaker. Typically inserted underneath the skin below one of the clavicles, a pacemaker communicates with the heart by a specialized wire(s) inserted through a nearby vein. It is able to make sure that heart rate does not become too slow by providing an electrical stimulus for the heart to beat. This is an action called "pacing." When heart rate is *not* too slow a pacemaker is able to recognize this and not pace. This is a process called "sensing." In its simplest terms this is what a pacemaker does.

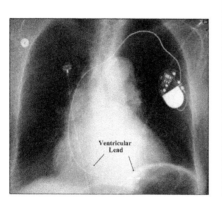
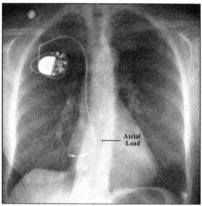

Pacemakers essentially come in two varieties, "single chamber" and "dual chamber." As the name implies, a single-chamber pacemaker only functions in one chamber of the heart. This can be accomplished with a single wire placed either in the atrium or ventricle. Which type of single-chamber pacemaker is used depends on what type of heart rhythm abnormality a patient has.

A pacemaker is able to ensure that a patient's heart rate will not become too slow by producing an _____ stimulus for the heart to beat.

In its simplest terms a pacemaker performs two functions called _____ and _____.

ELECTRICAL
PACING, SENSING

A dual-chamber pacemaker functions in two chambers of the heart, one chamber being an atrium and one a ventricle. This allows the normal sequence of beating, atrial contraction followed by ventricular contraction, to be maintained even in the face of heart block. Thus, a separate wire in each chamber is most often required to allow this function to occur.

Whether a single- or a dual-chamber pacemaker is used depends on the heart rhythm abnormality and the preference of the physician implanting the pacemaker.

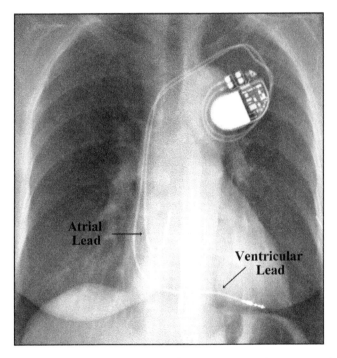

A dual-chamber pacemaker most often has two wires, one placed in the _____ and the other in the _____.

The normal sequence of _____ can be maintained with a dual-chamber pacemaker.

ATRIUM, VENTRICLE
CONTRACTION

Chapter 3

Pacemaker System and Cardiac Anatomy

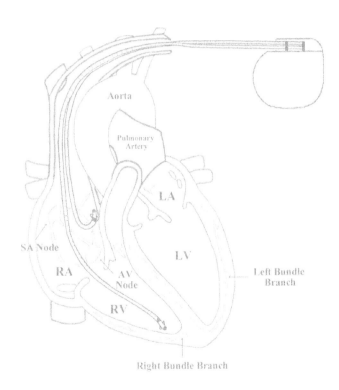

PACEMAKER SYSTEM AND CARDIAC ANATOMY

Pacemaker wires, or "leads," are inserted underneath the clavicle into a vein, through which they are advanced to the heart. The tip of a ventricular pacemaker lead is typically placed in the apex of the right ventricle (RV). This is near the right bundle branch (RBB) of the native conduction system. An atrial pacemaker lead tip is typically placed in the appendage of the right atrium (RA). Pacemaker leads are not implanted within the left atrium (LA) or left ventricle (LV) as they have the potential for causing a stroke. Rarely, pacemaker leads are attached to the outside surface of the heart during an open heart surgical procedure. In this case they may be placed on the surface of the left side of the heart.

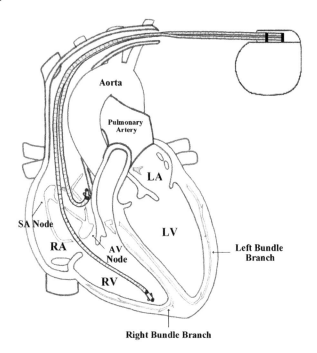

Atrial and ventricular pacemaker leads are typically placed in the _____ and the _____, respectively.

A pacemaker lead placed within the RV may be near the _____ _____ _____ of the native conduction system.

RA APPENDAGE, RV APEX
RIGHT BUNDLE BRANCH

Chapter 4

The Hardware

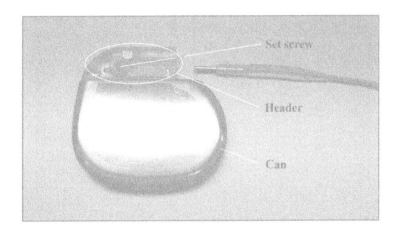

The Hardware

A complete permanent pacing system includes the pacemaker itself and the pacemaker lead(s). They may also be referred to as a "pacemaker or pulse generator" and "electrode(s)," respectively.

The Pacemaker Generator

The pacemaker is both the power source and the brains of the pacing system. As such, it contains a battery and electronic circuitry that perform these functions.

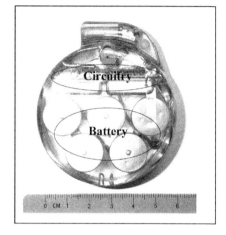

The Battery

Each pacemaker contains a battery whose lifetime varies depending on how much it is used to pace the heart. Typical longevities generally fall between 5 and 10 years. When the battery begins to wear down it does not suddenly quit, but rather shows signs over many months time that this is happening with changes in what is called the "magnet rate," or other rate indicators.

Placement of a magnet over a pacemaker causes it to pace at a rate that is predetermined by each pacemaker manufacturer, and regardless of the patient's own heart rhythm (in other words, it ignores the patient's own heart rhythm). This "magnet rate" changes when the battery begins to wear down. The battery alone cannot be exchanged, so a new pacemaker is used to replace one whose battery is worn.

A pacemaker contains both a _____ and _____ _____.

The pacemaker battery may last from _____ years.

BATTERY, ELECTRONIC CIRCUITRY
5 to 10

The Circuitry

The pacemaker's electronic circuitry contains the necessary elements for determining when and how the pacemaker system functions. These functions may be changed, or "programmed," even after the pacemaker is implanted within the body, through the use of a special computer called a "pacemaker programmer." Pacemakers have different functional abilities based on the sophistication of its circuitry.

Over the years both pacing battery and electronic circuit technology have improved, which has allowed the pacemaker generator to greatly diminish in size.

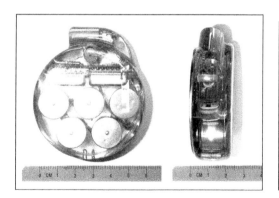 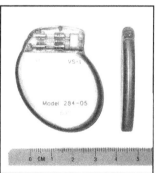

A pacemaker generator may be _____ to function in a different fashion.

A pacemaker generator's abilities are determined by its _____.

PROGRAMMED
CIRCUITRY

The "Header" and "Can"

In order for a pacemaker to communicate with the heart it needs to be connected to a pacemaker lead(s). At the top of each pacemaker generator is a structure called the "header." The header provides a hole for each pacemaker lead to be inserted. On the side of each header is a "set screw" that may be tightened to fix a lead in place, or loosened to allow a lead to be removed. Some pacemakers have two set screws for each pacemaker lead.

The metal casing of the pacemaker generator is called the "can." The can protects the battery and circuitry from fluids and most outside electrical/energy sources (this includes microwave ovens but possibly not cellular telephones operating very close to the pacemaker generator and specific hospital diagnostic and therapeutic equipment!). Because it is metal, the can may also function as a part of a pacemaker's pacing or sensing circuit.

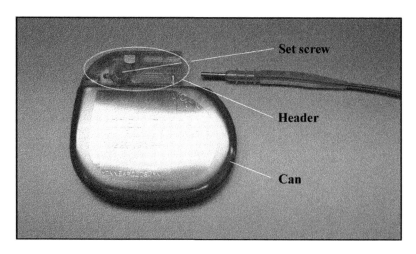

A pacemaker lead is inserted in a pacemaker generator at the _____ and held in place by tightening the _____.

The _____ is the metal casing that protects the pacemaker battery and circuitry from fluids and most external electrical sources.

HEADER, SET SCREW(S)
CAN

THE PACEMAKER LEAD

A pacemaker lead is essentially a flexible coiled metal wire, encased either in silicone rubber or polyurethane insulation, that transmits electrical signals between the heart and pacemaker. The insulation serves to direct electrical signals only along the wire and prevent them from traveling to places other than between the pacemaker and heart. The lead is a separate element from the pacemaker and is connected to it only after being implanted in the body. A pacemaker lead is typically between 45 and 58 cm in length.

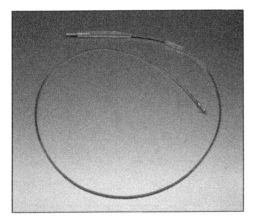
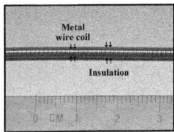

A pacemaker lead consists of a _____ metal wire encased by either silicone rubber or polyurethane _____.

The length of a typical pacemaker lead is between _____ and _____ in length.

COILED, INSULATION
45, 58 cm

Each pacemaker lead is classified by whether it is configured with one ("unipolar") or two ("bipolar") separate points of electrical contact within the heart. This is an important distinction, because the configuration affects the manner and characteristic of the electrical signals received from the heart and delivered to the pacemaker.

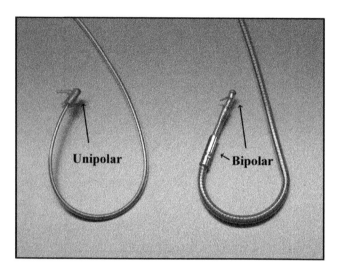

A bipolar pacemaker lead configuration has _____ points and a unipolar pacemaker lead configuration _____ point of contact within the heart.

TWO, ONE

Unipolar Versus Bipolar Configuration

In a unipolar configuration, the can of the pacemaker participates in the pacemaker circuit. Each pacing stimulus is delivered between the pacemaker lead tip and pacemaker can. Therefore not only may the heart be paced, but also rarely chest muscles underlying the pacemaker generator may be stimulated to contract. Electrical activity occurring anywhere between the can and the lead tip may be sensed and interpreted as a cardiac event. This includes the electrical signal generated by skeletal muscle (a situation called "myopotential oversensing") or cardiac electrical activity occurring in a heart chamber other than where the lead tip resides (a situation called "atrial or ventricular oversensing").

As opposed to a unipolar configuration, a bipolar configuration does not involve the pacemaker can in the pacemaker circuit. Instead a bipolar configuration utilizes the small window between the bipoles on the lead for pacing and sensing. This small window makes it extremely unlikely that skeletal muscle may be paced or that oversensing may occur.

There is also a difference in the appearance of a unipolar (large) versus a bipolar (small) pacing spike on the surface ECG. Examples of this may be seen in chapter 7 (*Pacing and Capture*).

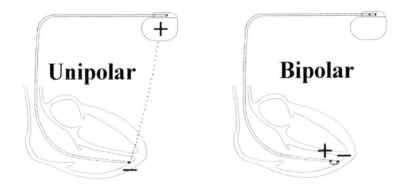

A _____ pacemaker lead configuration utilizes the pacemaker can in its circuit, while a _____ configuration does not.

A _____ pacemaker lead configuration is more likely to _____ and pace skeletal muscle.

UNIPOLAR, BIPOLAR
UNIPOLAR, OVERSENSE

Pacemaker leads may also be classified by their mechanism of attachment to the heart. "Active fixation" leads have a mechanism at their tip which helps keep the lead tip in place in the heart. Most commonly they are a "screw-in" type that actually screws into the heart wall. "Passive fixation" leads are commonly "tined" and hold onto muscular strands like a grappling hook. A lead tip without fixation may be used for a temporary pacing circumstance. It is not uncommon for a passive fixation lead tip to move (in technical terms, "dislodge") and cause a disruption in pacing and/or sensing function. It uncommonly happens that an active fixation lead tip may dislodge.

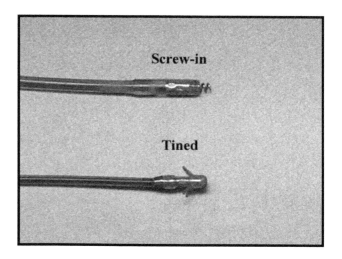

Screw-in pacemaker leads are types of _____ leads.

Passive fixation leads have _____ active mechanism for keeping their lead tip in place.

A pacemaker lead tip that has moved is said to have _____.

ACTIVE FIXATION
NO
DISLODGED

THE PACEMAKER PROGRAMMER

The pacemaker programmer is a specialized device used to communicate with and, if needed, change the manner in which a pacemaker functions. Communication may be established via telemetry when the pacemaker programmer's "head" is placed over the area where the pacemaker generator lies. Once telemetry is established, all of the functions of the pacemaker may be determined through a process called "interrogation" and displayed for review both on the screen of the programmer and on paper by having the programmer print the information. The programmer may also be used to perform certain tests that allow the performance of the pacemaker system to be evaluated.

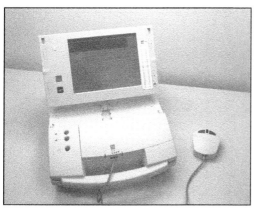
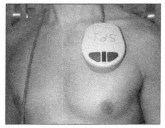

There are many different pacemaker manufacturers, all of whom have their own programmers that are specific to their own devices. In other words, a programmer from pacemaker company *A* cannot be used to communicate with a pacemaker from company *B*.

In order to determine how a pacemaker is set up to function, a pacemaker _____ may be used to _____ it and display the information on a screen.

Pacemaker programmers are _____ to the company that manufactured the pacemaker generator.

PROGRAMMER, INTERROGATE
SPECIFIC

Programmer Telemetry

After a pacemaker generator has been interrogated, all of its current programmed parameters are transmitted to the programmer via telemetry, where they are available to be printed and reviewed.

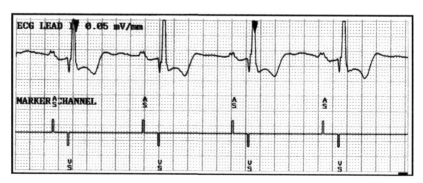

In addition pacemaker ECG rhythm strips may be printed from the programmer by attaching the programmer's ECG cables to the patient. Rhythm strips may be accompanied by annotations commonly referred to as "marker channels" beneath the ECG.

A pacemaker and programmer communicate via _____.

ECG _____ _____ may be printed from a pacemaker programmer.

TELEMETRY
RHYTHM STRIPS

Marker channels are also obtained from the pacemaker via telemetry and indicate what the pacemaker is doing in real time. They are an important aid for interpreting pacemaker ECG rhythms and will be used on occasion throughout the book.

Each marker channel annotation represents an atrial and ventricular event on the ECG as either being paced or sensed. The annotations differ slightly between pacemaker manufacturers, but convey the same information. For example, an atrial sensed event may be represented as "AS" or "P" (for P wave) and an atrial paced event as "AP" or "A." A ventricular sensed event may be represented as "VS" or "R" (for R wave) and a ventricular paced event as "VP" or "V." Both atrial and ventricular events are annotated for a dual-chamber pacemaker, while only atrial or ventricular events may be annotated for a single-chamber atrial or ventricular pacemaker, respectively.

Marker channels may also include numbers with the lettered annotations. They represent the time intervals between the events.

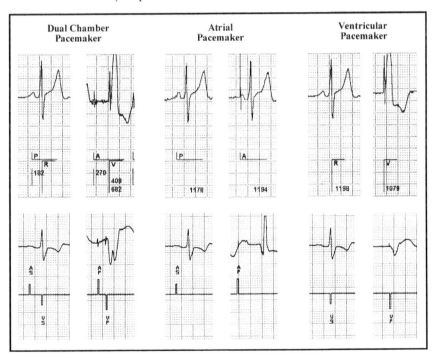

Marker channels are an annotation of atrial and/or ventricular _____ on an ECG rhythm strip.

EVENTS

An ECG rhythm strip may also be printed with a signal called an electrogram (EGM) that is recorded by the pacemaker and transmitted to the programmer by telemetry. An EGM represents the local electrical activity as recorded by a pacemaker lead tip in the heart. EGMs will be described in more detail in chapters 5 (*Electronics 101*) and 6 (*Sensing and Sensitivity*).

Other useful information that may be obtained from a pacemaker with telemetry includes counters that keep track of how much of the time a pacemaker is required to pace and sense and how often heart rate reaches certain levels.

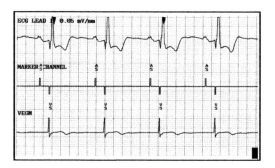

Initial Interrogation Report			Page 3
Atrial High Rate Episodes: 33			
Date/Time	Duration hh:mm:ss		Max Atrial Rate (bpm)
03/09/00 8:48 AM	:02	First	155
04/20/00 12:19 PM	:24	Fastest	>400
04/20/00 12:21 PM	:01:02	Longest	>400
04/20/00 1:46 PM	:06	Last	400
Ventricular High Rate Episodes: 56			
Date/Time	Duration hh:mm:ss		Max Vent. Rate (bpm)
02/11/00 3:10 PM	:01	First	183
04/20/00 11:02 AM	:01:08	Longest	>400
04/20/00 1:46 PM	:02	Fastest	>400
04/20/00 1:46 PM	:02	Last	>400
Pacing (% of total):		**Event Counters**	
AS - VS	0.1%	PVC singles	7,691
AS - VP	97.4%	PVC runs	1,377
AP - VS	< 0.1%	PAC runs	212
AP - VP	2.4%		

The electrical activity that is recorded locally to a pacemaker lead tip is referred to as an _____.

_____ may be used by a pacemaker to keep track of what amount of time that it is pacing and sensing.

EGM
COUNTERS

THE PACEMAKER MAGNET

The pacemaker magnet is a fairly strong magnet (typically 90 "gauss," or a good multiple of all of your refrigerator magnets combined!) used for evaluating both pacemaker pacing function and pacemaker battery status.

When a pacemaker magnet is placed over a pacemaker generator, it begins to pace at a fixed rate in an "asynchronous" mode, or "magnet mode." It does not sense! Another way of putting this is that it paces at a fixed rate regardless of whatever the patient's own heart rhythm is. Atrial and then ventricular pacing ensue at a fixed rate after magnet placement for dual-chamber pacemakers with both atrial and ventricular pacing function active. Single-chamber pacemakers pace at a fixed rate in whatever chamber that there is active

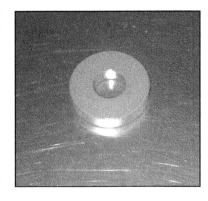

pacing function. Thus, the integrity of atrial and/or ventricular pacing can be quickly identified with magnet placement.

The fixed rate that a pacemaker paces at after magnet placement is termed the "magnet rate." Changes in the magnet rate (usually steps down in the fixed pacing rate, i.e., from 85 pulses per minute [ppm] to 75 ppm) over time are indicative of a pacemaker battery that is beginning to wear down. Magnet rate is set by each pacemaker manufacturer and is easily found in either the technical manual that comes with each new pacemaker generator, or in any of the reference guides published by each pacemaker manufacturer. Thus, knowing what a particular pacemaker generator's magnet rate is allows quick evaluation of the battery status with magnet placement.

Placement of a magnet on a pacemaker generator causes it to pace in an _____ manner and at a _____ rate.

A magnet rate that has changed may be indicative of a pacemaker _____ that is beginning to wear down.

ASYNCHRONOUS, FIXED
BATTERY

Chapter 5

Electronics 101

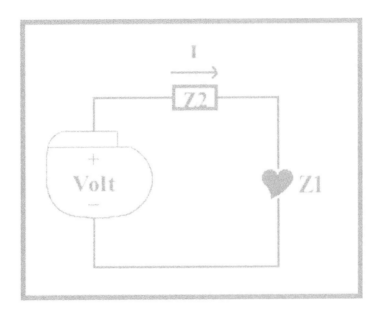

Electronics 101

In order to understand how a pacemaker interacts with the heart it is essential to know some basics of electric circuitry. Why? This knowledge becomes most useful when troubleshooting certain pacing system malfunctions. More on this to follow!

First, here are a few essential terms:

Voltage: The force by which electrical current is made to flow. Frequently described as a "voltage potential," it is created when positive and negative charges are separated. Units are called "volts" (V).

Current: The flow of charge past a given point per unit time. Units are "amperes" (A). Most commonly, the level of current in a pacemaker circuit is measured in 1/1000 of an ampere or "milliamperes" (mA).

Resistance: The opposition to the flow of electrical current. Its units are called "ohms" (Ω).

Energy: The product of [**voltage * current * time**]. The units of energy are "joules" (J). With regard to the heart, voltage and current occur over "milliseconds" (ms; 1/1000 of a second) and energy is on the order of "microjoules" (μJ; one millionth of a joule) in a pacemaker circuit.

_____ may be made to flow when a _____ potential is created.

Current flow is opposed by _____.

The product of [**voltage * current * time**] defines _____.

CURRENT, VOLTAGE
RESISTANCE
ENERGY

A basic electric circuit may typically consist of a voltage source and a resistor. The voltage source has a positive and a negative terminal which, when connected to both ends of the resistor, can cause current to flow across the circuit. The relationship between the voltage, current, and resistance may then be described by the equation, **V (voltage) = I (current; in Amps) * R (re-**

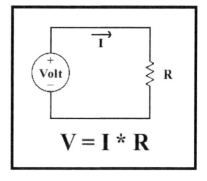

$$V = I * R$$

sistance). This is "Ohm's law." For example, if a circuit has a voltage of 10 V and resistance of 5 Ω, then by Ohm's law the current that may flow in the circuit is 2 A (10 V/5 Ω).

A different circuit can be created by connecting another resistor in parallel to the first. The combined resistance of the two is less than the value of either of them, and is equal to their product divided by their sum. As an example, the combined resistance of two 5-Ω resistors in parallel is 2.5 Ω ([5 5]/[5+5]). Thus by Ohm's law if the voltage is kept the same before and after the second resistor is applied in parallel, the total current (**It**) must increase to compensate for the decreased resistance. The current in the above example would then be 4 A (10 V/2.5 Ω).

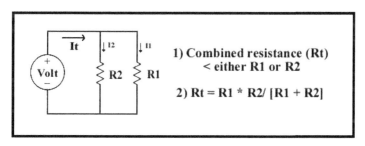

1) Combined resistance (Rt)
   < either R1 or R2

2) Rt = R1 * R2/ [R1 + R2]

The equation **V = I R** is called _____.

The combined resistance of two resistors in parallel is _____ than the value of either of them.

OHM'S LAW
LESS

Yet another type of circuit can be created when a second resistor is added in series with the first. The combined resistance is simply their sum. So, if two 5-Ω resistors are connected in series their combined resistance is 10 Ω (5+5)! By Ohm's law, if voltage is the same before and after the second resistor is added in series, then the current must decrease in order to compensate for the increased resistance. This would be 1 A for a 10-V source connected to two 5-Ω resistors in series (10/ [5 2] = 1).

If resistance is sufficiently large, then current flow will be negligible. The most extreme example of this is when there is a break in the circuit. Resistance then becomes infinitely large, and no current flows.

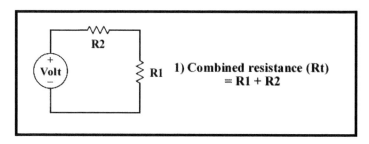

The combined resistance of resistors in series is their _____.

If resistance is infinitely large, then no _____ will flow.

The voltage of a circuit in which a 10-A current flows to two 5-Ω resistors connected in parallel is _____.

The voltage of a circuit in which a 10-A current flows to two 5-Ω resistors connected in series is _____.

SUM
CURRENT
25 V (10 A 2.5 Ω)
100 V (10 A 10 Ω)

Resistance does not include all of the forces opposing current flow. A term used to describe this total opposition to current flow, and more applicable to a true pacemaker circuit, is "impedance." Its units are also Ω and it is typically represented in electrical terms by a capital "Z." Thus, the equation relating voltage, impedance, and current becomes $V = Z * I$. As with resistance, impedance sources in series and parallel are combined similarly to calculate their combined total impedance.

For the pacemaker circuit, impedance can be measured automatically by a pacemaker programmer and is termed "lead impedance." It may range from approximately 300 to 1200 Ω, depending on the type of pacemaker lead used, and tends to stay fairly constant over time.

Now let us apply all of this theory to the heart! The pacemaker can represent a voltage source and the heart an impedance source (Z_1). A pacemaker lead and the body tissue itself represent the wiring connecting the heart to the pacemaker. The pacemaker lead and body tissue also add impedance in series to the circuit (Z_2). In this configuration, current may flow across the circuit and stimulate the heart, thus causing it to beat!

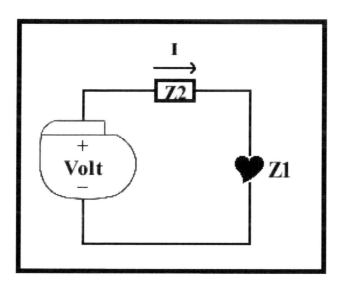

The total opposition to current flow in a pacemaker circuit may be referred to as _____.

Lead impedance may typically be between _____ and _____.

LEAD IMPEDANCE
300, 1200 Ω

The lead impedance also becomes a useful piece of information, as dramatic changes in it may indicate a problem in the pacemaker circuit. For example, if a lead impedance over many years is about 1100 Ω, but a new measurement reveals it to be 500 Ω, this is cause for concern. Although the new value is within the range of normal, it represents a significant change and may suggest a pacemaker lead insulation break. This is how:

When an insulation break occurs in the pacemaker lead, a path is created that allows current to flow parallel to the heart. The impedance of this new circuit decreases. If voltage is to remain constant, an increased current drain occurs that can prematurely deplete the pacemaker battery. Also, if there is skeletal muscle along the new path it can be stimulated by the pacemaker output.

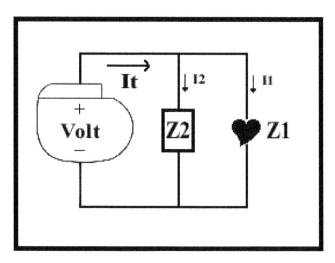

A pacemaker lead insulation break may cause current to flow _____ to the heart, lead impedance to _____, and _____ pacemaker battery depletion.

PARALLEL, DECREASE, PREMATURE

Conversely, a significant increase in lead impedance may suggest a pacemaker lead fracture. A pacemaker lead fracture may cause an intermittent or a complete break in the circuit without compromising the lead insulation. The break adds significant impedance to current flow in series with the heart that may be of such magnitude so as to prevent the heart from being stimulated. Of note, a lead fracture is not the only cause of an increased lead impedance. Another cause includes a loose set screw holding the lead in the pacemaker.

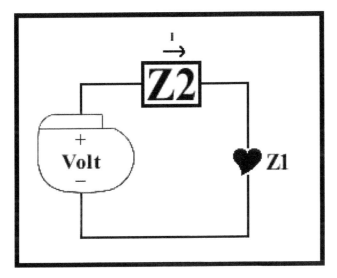

A pacemaker lead fracture may cause lead impedance to _____.

A loose _____ _____ may also cause an increased lead impedance.

INCREASE
SET SCREW

The heart itself can also act as a voltage source (on the order of millivolts [mV]; 1/1000 of a volt). When it beats, an electrical signal spreads across its surface and to the pacemaker lead. Current can then flow back to the pacemaker where it can arrive at the pacemaker's sensing circuit.

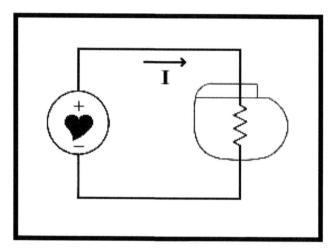

Electrical activity from the heart may cause _____ to flow back to the pacemaker.

The size of the voltage potential from the heart is on the order of _____.

CURRENT
MILLIVOLTS (mV)

THE ELECTROGRAM

Whereas a surface ECG represents a summation of all cardiac electrical activity as seen on the body surface, an electrogram (EGM) represents the local cardiac electrical activity at a pacemaker lead tip within the heart. If a pacemaker lead tip is located in the atrium, then an atrial EGM (AEGM) is recorded. The main deflection on an AEGM is referred to as a "P wave." If a pacemaker lead tip is located in the ventricle then a ventricular EGM (VEGM) is recorded. The main deflection on a VEGM is referred to as an "R wave." The P and R waves on their respective EGMs correspond roughly in time to the P and R waves on the surface ECG.

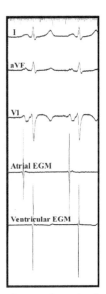

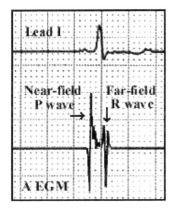

An EGM may also record an electrical component originating a distance away from the lead tip. This component is termed the "far-field" signal. The signal originating at the lead tip is called the "near-field signal." For example, an AEGM may have a ventricular component ("far-field R wave") after the atrial component ("near-field P wave"). The pacemaker needs to be able to ignore the far-field component.

An _____ is the term used to describe the electrical signal as recorded from within the heart.

The _____ signal refers to the component recorded on an EMG that originates a distance away from the pacemaker lead tip.

The _____ signal describes the EGM electrical component originating at the pacemaker lead tip.

EGM
FAR-FIELD
NEAR-FIELD

Chapter 6

Sensing and Sensitivity

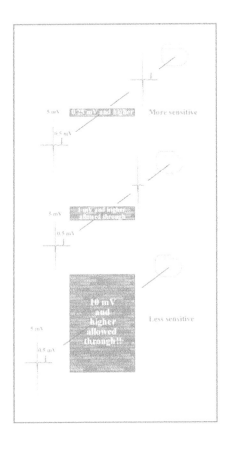

SENSING AND SENSITIVITY

Each component of an electrogram (EGM) is not necessarily seen or "sensed" by the pacemaker. One way that it determines which signal component may be sensed is by setting a minimum height, measured in "millivolts" (mV) which each component has to at least reach before the pacemaker sensing circuitry may recognize it. This minimum height is called the "sensitivity." A small sensitivity setting makes it more likely that a signal component will measure up to the smaller minimum height (i.e., the pacemaker is more sensitive). A larger sensitivity setting makes it less likely that a signal component will measure up to the larger minimum height (i.e., the pacemaker is less sensitive).

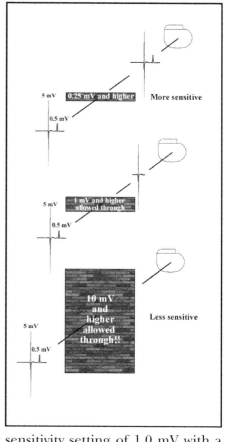

For example, a pacemaker sensitivity setting of 1.0 mV with a near-field P wave of 5 mV and a far-field R wave of 0.5 mV on an atrial EGM (AEGM) will allow a pacemaker to sense the P wave and ignore the far-field R wave. If the sensitivity setting is increased to 10 mV (pacemaker made less sensitive), then neither the P or R wave will be sensed because each is not tall enough. On the other hand, if the sensitivity setting is decreased to 0.25 mV (pacemaker made more sensitive) then both P and R wave may be sensed because both are tall enough.

The R wave amplitude on a ventricular EGM (VEGM) is typically greater than the P wave amplitude on an AEGM, and is on the order of 5 to 25 mV. P wave amplitude on an AEGM is usually between 1.5 and 5 mV. As such, sensitivity settings for a ventricular pacemaker are higher (less sensitive) than that for an atrial pacemaker (more sensitive). Also, there are separate sensitivity settings for the atrial and ventricular leads of a dual-chamber pacing system because of this disparity in EGM size. They help the pacemaker differentiate what is truly ventricular in origin on a VEGM, and what is truly atrial in origin on an AEGM. The pacemaker has other means to aid in this differentiation that will be covered in Section II.

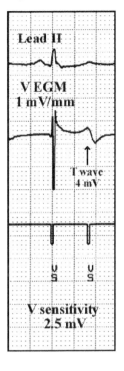

The pacemaker can rarely at times be fooled. Such an example is that of "T wave oversensing." The T wave can appear on a VEGM and be of such amplitude that the pacemaker recognizes it as an R wave.

The minimum height that an EGM component needs to be in order that it may be sensed is the _____.

Increasing the sensitivity setting makes a pacemaker _____ sensitive.

In order to make a pacemaker more sensitive the sensitivity setting is _____.

SENSITIVITY
LESS
DECREASED

Chapter 7

Pacing and Capture

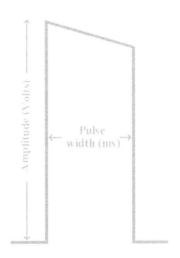

PACING AND CAPTURE

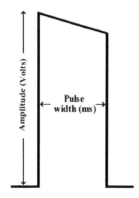

In order to make the heart beat, the pacemaker produces an electrical pacing stimulus. The pacing stimulus, also called "spike," "impulse," or "output," can be described in terms of its amplitude (most commonly volts [V]) and pulse width (milliseconds [ms]). Both of these parameters may be programmed. Whether a stimulus actually makes the heart beat depends on a few factors:

Does the stimulus occur at a time when the heart is excitable (i.e., not in refractory)?

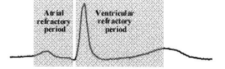

Is the stimulus of sufficient energy such that enough cardiac muscle cells are stimulated to reach threshold and initiate a depolarization wavefront?

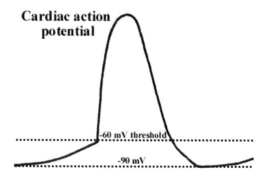

If both of these criteria are met then the heart chamber in which the stimulus is delivered may beat, a process otherwise called "capture."

A pacemaker stimulus may be described by both its _____ in volts and its _____ _____ in milliseconds (ms).

The process of causing the heart to beat in response to a pacing stimulus is called _____.

AMPLITUDE, PULSE WIDTH
CAPTURE

Ventricular capture is usually easy to distinguish, as the captured complex following a ventricular pacing spike differs dramatically from the native complex. This is because it may be wider in duration and has a left bundle branch block (LBBB) morphology. Why does it have an LBBB morphology?

Recall that the tip of the ventricular pacing lead most commonly sits in the right ventricle, which is close to the right bundle branch of the native conduction system. Therefore, with ventricular pacing the left bundle branch gets activated later and produces an LBBB complex.

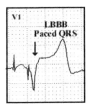 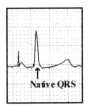

Should a ventricular captured beat display a right bundle branch block (RBBB) morphology, this may be cause for concern. The ventricular pacing lead tip may have penetrated into the left ventricle, a process called "perforation." This requires the lead to be pulled back because a clot can form on the pacing lead and cause a stroke, or because the lead can move even further and exit the heart! The other situation where an RBBB captured beat may occur, and does not require correction, is from a ventricular pacing lead implanted on the surface of the left ventricle in an open heart surgical procedure, or in a "bi-ventricular" pacing system.

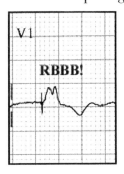

A captured ventricular beat should have an _____ morphology.

Ventricular lead perforation to the left ventricle is one cause of an _____ morphology paced ventricular beat.

LBBB
RBBB

A ventricular pacing spike may occur at a time when the native conduction system is early in activating the ventricles. This may cause the ventricles to contract from a combination of both native and pacemaker stimulation. The resultant ventricular beat is called a "fusion beat." A fusion beat may appear in various forms depending on whether native or pacemaker activation predominates. Fusion beats are a normal occurrence.

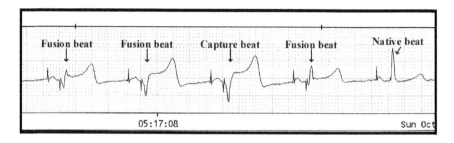

A fusion beat results from a combination of _____ and _____ activation.

The various forms of fusion beats occur depending on whether native or pacemaker activation _____.

Fusion beats may occur _____.

NATIVE, PACEMAKER
PREDOMINATES
NORMALLY

Atrial capture is determined on the ECG by noting a P wave after each atrial pacing spike. With normal native conduction to the ventricles a QRS may follow. This is an important sign because P waves are occasionally not readily seen after atrial pacing spikes but the native ventricular complexes associated with each unseen P wave are. In this case the native ventricular complexes are indicative of atrial capture.

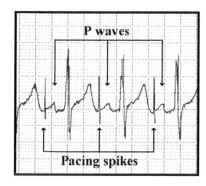
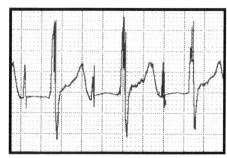

For dual-chamber pacemakers where a ventricular pacing spike follows each atrial pacing spike atrial capture may be difficult to see, even on a 12-lead ECG.

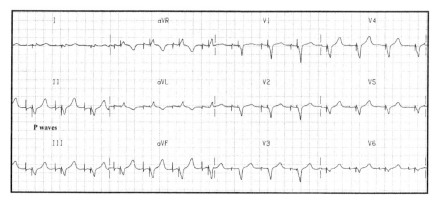

A P wave following each atrial pacing spike is indicative of _____ _____.

Occasionally a _____ may not be easily seen after an atrial pacing spike.

ATRIAL CAPTURE
P WAVE

Atrial capture is not the only feature of a pacing system that can be difficult to recognize on a surface ECG. The pacing spikes themselves can be invisible in a bipolar configuration. In this situation their presence may be noted with marker channels.

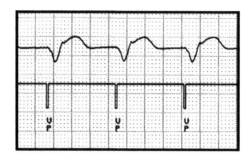

This is not always the case for a bipolar pacing configuration. Unipolar pacing spikes do not present such a problem, as they are larger than bipolar pacing spikes and are readily seen on the surface ECG.

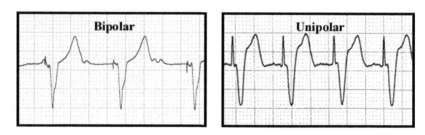

_____ pacing spikes may not be seen on a surface ECG.

_____ _____ may help identify unseen pacing spikes.

_____ pacing spikes are typically _____ than _____ pacing spikes.

BIPOLAR
MARKER CHANNELS
UNIPOLAR, LARGER, BIPOLAR

Chapter 8

Rate Versus Interval

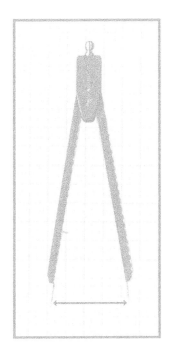

RATE VERSUS INTERVAL

Because most pacemaker timing cycles are described in terms of an interval, in milliseconds (ms), the ability to convert a given rate to its corresponding interval is quite helpful. This conversion is done simply with the following formula:

$$\text{INTERVAL (ms)} = \frac{60,000}{\text{RATE (pulses or beats per minute [bpm])}}$$

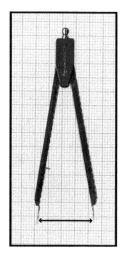

For example, the corresponding interval for a pacemaker rate of 70 bpm is 857 ms (60,000 ÷ 70).

In practice this conversion allows easy measurement of any pacemaker rate on an ECG grid with a pair of calipers (recall that each large box on a standard ECG grid equals 200 ms, and that there are five 40-ms boxes for each large box).

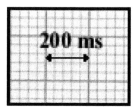

Comparisons between two rates and/or their corresponding intervals will be done frequently throughout the book. It is important to understand the difference between comparing the two. For example, one rate being *less than* the second has a corresponding interval that is *greater than* that of the faster rate, i.e.:

60 bpm < 70 bpm
vs.
1000 ms > 857 ms

To convert a given rate, in bpm, to an interval, in ms, you divide ＿＿＿＿＿ by the＿＿＿＿＿.

Each small box on a standard ECG grid equals ＿＿＿＿＿.

The corresponding interval for a heart rate of 80 bpm is ＿＿＿＿＿ than that for a heart rate of 50 bpm.

60,000, RATE
40 ms
LESS

Chapter 9

The Code and Mode

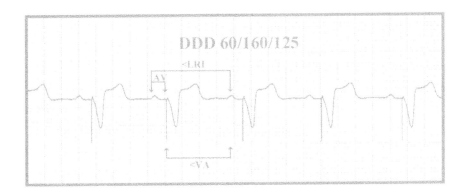

The Code and Mode

Pacemaker function is described by a universally accepted code devised by the North American and British pacing societies. The code provides for a description of pacemaker pacing and sensing function using a five-letter sequence. It is this sequence that is referred to as the "pacemaker mode." In practice, only the first three- or four-letter positions are commonly used to describe bradycardia pacing function (i.e., "DDD" or "VVIR").

The first letter position in the code describes the pacing capabilities:

A Paces Atrium
V Paces Ventricle
D Dual (Paces Atrium and Ventricle)
O None

The second letter position describes the sensing capabilities:

A Senses Atrium
V Senses Ventricle
D Dual (Senses Atrium and Ventricle)
O None

Pacemaker pacing and sensing function are described by a _____ whose letter sequence is referred to as the pacemaker _____.

CODE, MODE

The third letter position describes the response to sensing:

I Inhibits Pacing (i.e., don't want to pace into a chamber where a sensed event is occurring)

T Triggers Pacing (i.e., want to pace into a chamber where a sensed event is occurring)

D Inhibits and Triggers Pacing*

O None

The letter "I" in the third position of the pacemaker code refers to a pacemaker that _____ pacing in response to a sensed event.

Atrial sensing with the letter "D" in the third position of the pacemaker code will _____ atrial pacing and may trigger _____ _____ to occur a short period of time later.

INHIBITS
INHIBIT, VENTRICULAR PACING

The fourth letter position describes the presence of "rate modulation":

R Rate Modulating

O None

Rate modulation refers to the ability of the pacemaker to increase the rate of pacing on its own. The manner that the pacemaker does this is by having its own special sensors measure such things as vibration or minute ventilation (volume of air moved in 1 minute's time). The pacemaker uses these measurements as a determination of at least how fast heart rate should be. This rate is termed the "sensor indicated rate."

Rate modulation is typically used when a patient's heart will not appropriately increase its own rate with exertion or stress. This intrinsic inability to increase heart rate is called "chronotropic incompetence." Use of rate modulation also demands setting an upper limit on how fast the heart may be paced.

---

*This requires some further explanation. Only dual-chamber pacemakers may have this function. Atrial and ventricular sensing inhibit pacing in their respective chambers. Atrial sensing may also trigger ventricular pacing to occur a short period of time after it unless ventricular sensing occurs to inhibit it. Ventricular sensing may also inhibit atrial pacing in addition to ventricular pacing under circumstances where the pacemaker interprets the sensed event to be an event called a premature ventricular contraction (PVC).

The fifth position reflects recent revisions of the code and indicates the presence of "multisite" pacing (i.e., two atrial and/or ventricular leads).

A Atrium
V Ventricle
D Dual (A+V)
O None

Because recent advances in the area of multisite pacing have not fully defined the utility of these pacing modalities this topic will not be covered save references to "bi-ventricular" pacing in Chapter 17 and Section IV.

The presence of rate modulation is described by the _____ position in the code.

The _____ _____ _____ refers to at least how fast rate should be as determined by rate modulation.

Chronotropic incompetence refers to the inability of the heart to appropriately _____ its own rate with exertion or stress.

FOURTH
SENSOR INDICATED RATE
INCREASE

Putting this all together, a "DDD" mode describes a pacemaker mode with the ability to both pace and sense in the atrium and ventricle, and with both an inhibiting and triggering response to sensed events. "VVIR" describes a mode with ventricular pacing and sensing, inhibition of ventricular pacing as a response to ventricular sensing, and rate modulating function.

The first, second, and third positions in the pacemaker code, respectively, describe the pacemaker _____, _____, and _____ _____ functions.

A pacemaker with the ability to increase the pacing rate on its own is said to be _____ _____.

The three-letter sequence that describes a pacemaker mode with the ability to pace and sense in the atrium and with inhibition of atrial pacing in response to atrial sensing is _____.

PACING, SENSING, SENSING RESPONSE
RATE MODULATING
AAI

It is not enough to describe the pacemaker mode in order to understand how a pacemaker may function. There are many parameters that may be manipulated or "programmed" and will impact on function. Frequently, however, it is sufficient to know a select few parameters in addition to the pacemaker mode in order to read a pacemaker ECG rhythm strip. These parameters include the:

1) **Lower rate**. *The slowest that the pacemaker will allow heart rate to become.* Units are "pulses per minute" (ppm). Its corresponding interval is the "lower rate interval" (**LRI**). The interval unit is the "millisecond" (ms).
2) **Atrioventricular (AV) interval**. *The interval after an atrial event that the pacemaker will wait for a ventricular event to occur in a dual-chamber pacemaker.* Units are in ms.
3) **Upper rate limit (URL)**. *How fast the pacemaker will allow the heart to be paced.* Units are also ppm. Its corresponding interval, in ms, is the "upper rate interval" (**URI**).

The fastest and slowest that a pacemaker will pace the heart are, respectively, described by the _____ and the _____ _____.

URL, LOWER RATE

A commonly used convention may be used to summarize these parameters along with the pacemaker mode. For example, for single-chamber pacemakers:

Mode   lower rate/URL (if rate modulating)

. . . and for dual-chamber pacemakers:

Mode   lower rate/AV interval/URL

Thus, the annotation "**VVI 60**" denotes a pacemaker programmed to the VVI mode with a lower rate of 60 ppm, "**VVIR 60/120**" denotes a pacemaker programmed to the VVIR mode with a lower rate and URL of 60 and 120 ppm, respectively, and "**DDD 50/150/ 110**" denotes a pacemaker programmed to the DDD mode with a lower rate of 50 ppm, an AV interval of 150 ms, and a URL of 110 ppm. This convention will be used on all ECG rhythm strips to follow.

Now that the pacing basics and annotation of mode and pacing parameters have been covered its time to learn the pacing modes in detail. There are many different combinations of pacing and sensing, but only the most common of the modes will follow. Knowing them likely covers greater than 99% of all active pacing modes found in clinical practice.

A pacemaker programmed to the AAIR mode with a lower and upper rate of 60 and 130 ppm, respectively, may be annotated _____ _____.

AAIR 60/130

Section II

The Modes

Chapter 10

VVI Pacing

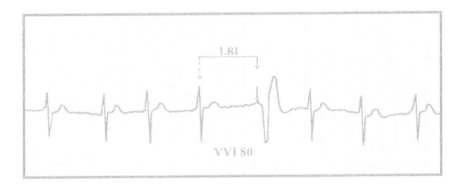

VVI PACING

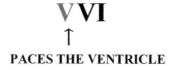

PACES THE VENTRICLE

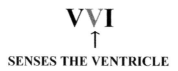

SENSES THE VENTRICLE

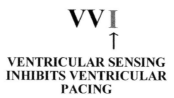

**VENTRICULAR SENSING
INHIBITS VENTRICULAR
PACING**

VVI PACING

The earliest form of permanent pacing was VOO! Shortly thereafter, pacemaker technology included reliable sensing circuitry and VVI pacing was born.

VVI pacing is now the most frequently prescribed pacing mode worldwide. This is likely so because the device is easier to implant, the ECGs are easier to interpret, and the pacing system is less expensive than a dual-chamber system. As an alternative to dual-chamber pacing, ventricular pacing can provide an increased pacing rate with exertion with the addition of rate modulation (VVIR).

It is very important to have a firm handle on interpreting this pacing mode, as the other modes build on its basic principles and only become more difficult to understand!

_____ pacing is the most frequently used mode of pacing worldwide.

VVI

VVI Timing

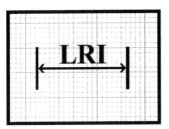

The basic timing cycle of a VVI pacemaker is the lower rate interval (LRI). This is the period of time that the pacemaker will wait to see if an R wave will occur before pacing the ventricle.

The LRI consist of two portions, the ventricular refractory period (VRP), and the alert period. The VRP is initiated at the start of the LRI with each sensed or paced event. It is a period during which pacemaker timing will not be affected by events that occur within it (i.e., no sensing with initiation of a new LRI!). The alert period follows and is the interval during which sensing can occur, inhibit pacing, and initiate a new LRI.

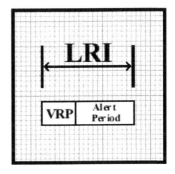

The VRP serves mostly to prevent the T wave of each QRS complex from being sensed.

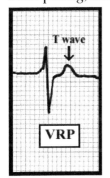

The basic timing cycle of a VVI pacemaker is the _____.

Events that occur during the VRP will not be _____ and initiate a new _____.

LRI
SENSED, LRI

A new LRI begins each time that a sensed or paced event occurs. The timing of each LRI subsequently ends when the next sensed or paced event happens. Thus, one of two things can happen after the initiation of each LRI. Either sensing occurs before the completion of the LRI, inhibits pacing, and starts a new LRI, or sensing does not occur before completion of the LRI, which elicits a pacemaker output and starts a new LRI.

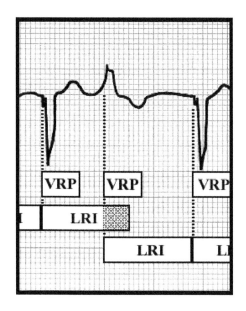

Patients frequently display a predominant pattern of pacing depending on how fast their own heart rate is. When the heart rate is predominantly faster than the pacemaker lower rate, a sensed pattern predominates, while with a heart rate slower than the pacemaker lower rate a paced pattern predominates.

A sensed or paced event starts a new _____.

If an R wave occurs faster than the lower rate it can be _____, _____ pacing, and _____ a new LRI.

LRI
SENSED, INHIBIT, START

When the Ventricular Rate is Faster Than the Lower Rate

A VVI pacemaker will sense "R waves" occurring after the VRP when the native ventricular rate is greater than the lower rate of the pacemaker. This is because each R wave occurs prior to completion of the LRI that started before it. On occasion, the LRI may pass without an R wave happening, so that the pacemaker needs to pace.

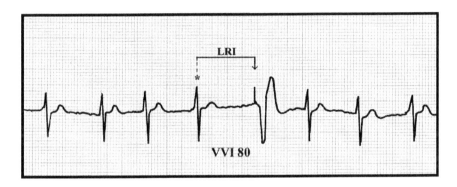

The name of the ventricular signal that the VVI pacemaker looks to sense is the _____ _____.

When the native ventricular rate is predominantly faster than the programmed lower rate a VVI pacemaker will predominantly _____ .

The LRI (in ms) is equal to _____ divided by the lower rate (in pulses per minute [ppm]).

R WAVE
SENSE
60,000

HYSTERESIS

Many VVI pacemakers have a rate function called "hysteresis."* "Positive" hysteresis can add an additional period of time for the pacemaker to wait and see if a native R wave will occur before pacing. In this application it can occur only after an R wave is sensed and does not occur after a paced event. The hysteresis rate is less than the lower rate. In this manner the principal purpose of hysteresis is to allow the patient to have his or her own underlying rhythm as much as possible. This can help conserve the pacemaker's battery life.

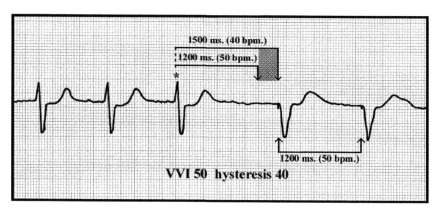

VVI 50 hysteresis 40

The positive hysteresis rate is _____ than the lower rate, and occurs only after a _____ ventricular event.

For example, if lower rate is 50 ppm (1200 ms) and hysteresis rate is 40 ppm (1500 ms), the pacemaker will wait _____ _____ after a sensed R wave before pacing the ventricle.

The less a pacemaker needs to pace then the _____ its battery life.

LESS, SENSED
1500 ms
LONGER

*This example features the most commonly encountered form of hysteresis; a hysteresis interval that is longer than the LRI. The hysteresis interval in other applications may be shorter than the LRI (see page 188, Pacing for Syncope). Because of these alternate applications hysteresis may be referred to as either being "positive" or "negative" depending on whether the hysteresis interval is longer or shorter than the programmed LRI.

When the Ventricular Rate is Slower Than the Lower Rate

A VVI pacemaker will pace at the lower programmed rate when the native ventricular rate is slower. This happens because each LRI completes timing before an R wave occurs. If an R wave is sensed, a VVI pacemaker will not pace until the LRI has completed timing.

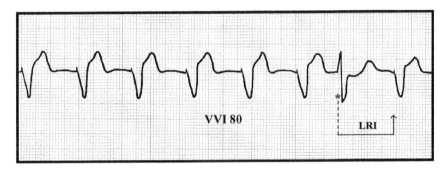

A ventricular heart rate that is slower than the lower rate will cause a VVI pacemaker to _____ at the lower rate.

A sensed R wave occurring before the LRI has completed will _____ ventricular pacing for that cycle and start timing of a new LRI.

PACE
INHIBIT

When the pacemaker is turned off and there is no native ventricular rhythm (i.e., the patient would not live), or it is sufficiently slow such that there are significant symptoms, then the patient is said to be "pacemaker dependent."

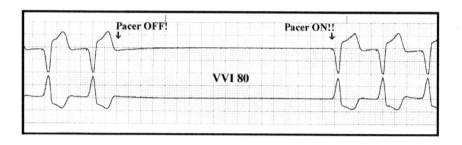

Patients who rely on their pacemaker to live are said to be _____ _____.

PACEMAKER DEPENDENT

Note: Pacemaker dependency can apply to any mode of active pacing and not just VVI!!

As a rule, one should not suddenly turn off pacing to determine if there is an underlying rhythm. This may likely result in a significant pause before an underlying rhythm, if present, returns. Turning the rate down slowly will generally avoid this problem.

RATE MODULATION

A VVIR pacemaker can progressively pace faster than the lower rate, but no more than the upper sensor rate limit, when it determines that heart rate needs to increase. This typically occurs with exercise in patients that cannot increase their own heart rate (see chronotropic incompetence, page 67). The amount of rate increase is determined by how much exertion the pacemaker thinks the patient is performing. This increased pacing rate is sometimes referred to as the "sensor indicated rate." When exertion has stopped the pacemaker will progressively decrease the paced rate down to the lower rate.

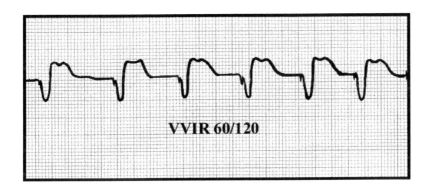

VVIR 60/120

The name for the condition whereby a person cannot increase their heart rate is _____ _____.

A VVIR pacemaker can pace _____ than the lower rate.

The _____ _____ is how fast above the lower rate that a rate modulating pacemaker determines pacing should be.

CHRONOTROPIC INCOMPETENCE
FASTER
SENSOR INDICATED RATE

Note: Many pacemakers have a sensor that uses vibration as a means of determining how much a person is exerting. This can at times inappropriately increase the paced rate when the person is not exercising (e.g., driving on a bumpy road or sitting on a riding lawn mower).

Magnet Mode (VOO)

Placement of a magnet on a VVI(R) pacemaker will cause it to pace the ventricle asynchronously at the magnet rate regardless of the underlying rhythm. It *does not sense!* If the native rhythm is slower than magnet rate then ventricular capture will occur at the magnet rate.

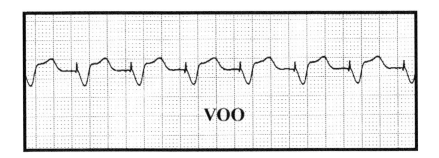

VOO pacing occurs when a _____ is placed on a pacemaker in the VVI(R) mode.

Pacing without _____ is also called "asynchronous" pacing.

MAGNET
SENSING

When the ventricular rate is faster than magnet rate periods of ventricular capture, fusion, or functional noncapture (pacing into native refractory periods, i.e., into a native R or T wave) may be seen.

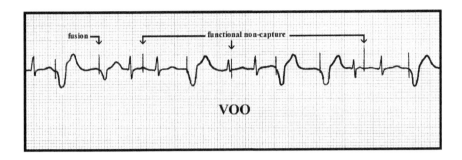

_____ is the name for the process that results in a QRS complex showing pacing capture and native conduction.

The magnet rate can change over time, which is indicative of a pacemaker _____ that is beginning to wear down. This is true of all pacing modes.

FUSION
BATTERY

Chapter 11

AAI Pacing

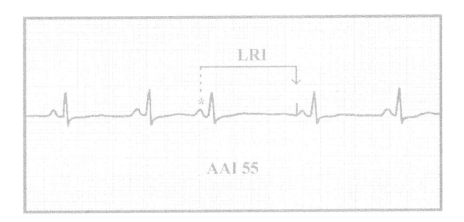

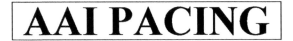

AAI PACING

A AI
↑
PACES THE ATRIUM

AAI
↑
SENSES THE ATRIUM

AAI
↑
ATRIAL SENSING INHIBITS
ATRIAL PACING

AAI PACING

AAI pacing is a much less commonly used mode of pacing for multiple reasons. It is contraindicated in atrial fibrillation (AF) and heart block. There is also a concern (not necessarily established) of heart block developing over time after implantation. Rhythm strips with AAI pacing can be slightly more difficult to interpret than those with VVI pacing, especially when the pacing spike is not readily seen (i.e., "is this native rhythm or AAI pacing?").

On the plus side, AAI pacing maintains the normal sequence of atrioventricular (AV) activation and may be associated with improved patient longevity when compared with VVI pacing.

AAI pacing is contraindicated in _____ and _____.

AF, HEART BLOCK

AAI TIMING

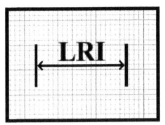

The basic timing cycle of an AAI pacemaker is the lower rate interval (LRI). This is the period of time that the pacemaker will wait to see if a P wave will occur before pacing the atrium.

The LRI consist of two portions, the atrial refractory period (ARP), and the alert period. The ARP is initiated at the start of the LRI with each sensed or paced event. It is a period during which pacemaker timing will not be affected by events that occur within it (i.e., no sensing with initiation of a new LRI!). The alert period follows and is the interval during which sensing can occur, inhibit pacing, and initiate a new LRI.

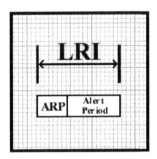

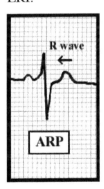

The ARP serves to prevent the far-field R wave from being sensed.

The basic timing cycle of an AAI pacemaker is the _____.

Events that occur during the _____ will not be _____ and initiate a new LRI.

LRI
ARP, SENSED

A new LRI begins each time that a sensed or paced event occurs. The timing of each LRI subsequently ends when the next sensed or paced event happens. Thus, one of two things can happen after the initiation of each LRI. Either sensing occurs before the completion of the LRI, inhibits pacing, and starts a new LRI, or sensing does not occur before completion of the LRI, which elicits a pacemaker output and starts a new LRI. Which sequence occurs is dependent on how fast the patient's own heart rate is.

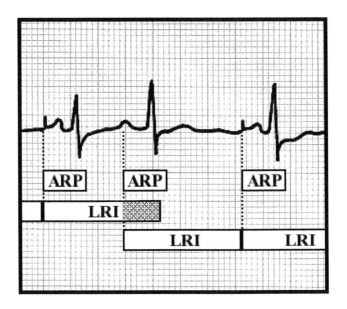

A sensed or paced event starts a new _____.

If a P wave occurs faster than the lower rate it can be _____, _____ pacing, and _____ a new LRI.

LRI
SENSED, INHIBIT, START

When the Atrial Rate is Faster Than the Lower Rate

An AAI pacemaker will predominantly sense when the native atrial rate is predominantly faster. If the LRI completes a cycle without sensing a "P wave" after the ARP then it will pace the atrium. As in the VVI mode, hysteresis can be employed. This will occur after sensing P waves only.

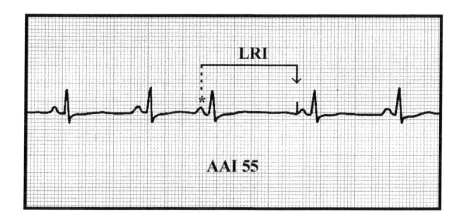

Sensing a _____ _____ outside the ARP will inhibit atrial pacing for that cycle and begin timing of a new LRI.

After an LRI in which no P waves are sensed an AAI pacemaker will _____ the _____.

Positive hysteresis in an AAI pacemaker can occur after _____ a P wave and at a rate that is _____ than lower rate.

P WAVE
PACE, ATRIUM
SENSING, SLOWER

When the Atrial Rate is Slower Than the Lower Rate

An AAI pacemaker will pace at the lower rate when the native atrial rate is slower. The pacemaker will not pace until the LRI has timed out after a sensed P wave.

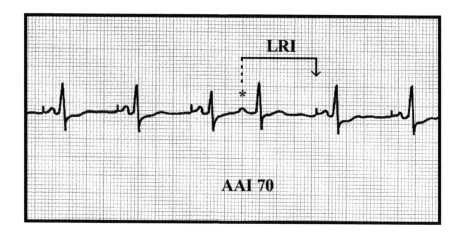

An atrial rate that is _____ than the lower rate will cause the AAI pacemaker to _____ at the lower rate.

A sensed P wave occurring before the _____ has completed will inhibit pacing for that cycle and start timing of a new _____.

SLOWER, PACE
LRI, LRI

RATE MODULATION

Rate modulation in an AAIR pacemaker will increase the atrial pacing rate with exertion in a chronotropically incompetent patient. This provides both a physiologic heart rate response and sequence of AV activation.

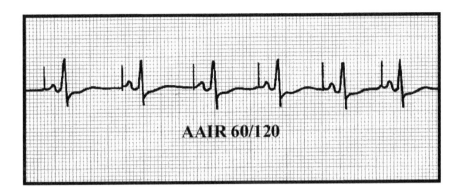

AAIR 60/120

An atrial pacemaker that increases its pacing rate above the lower rate is utilizing _____ _____.

Atrial pacing is said to be _____ because it maintains the normal AV activation sequence.

RATE MODULATION
PHYSIOLOGIC

Magnet Mode (AOO)

Placement of a magnet on an AAI(R) pacemaker will cause it to pace the atrium asynchronously at the magnet rate regardless of the underlying rhythm. *It does not sense!* If the native atrial rate is slower than the magnet rate, then atrial capture at the magnet rate occurs.

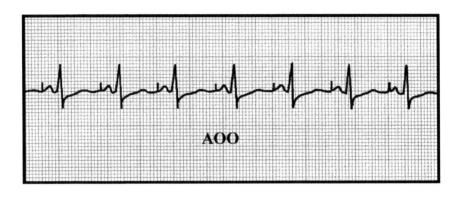

_____ pacing occurs when a magnet is placed on a pacemaker in the AAI(R) mode.

With AOO pacing there is no _____.

AOO
SENSING

When the native atrial rate is faster than the magnet rate periods of atrial capture or functional noncapture (pacing into native refractory periods) may be seen. Fusion is virtually impossible to determine with atrial pacing. The term should be reserved for reference to occurrences with ventricular pacing.

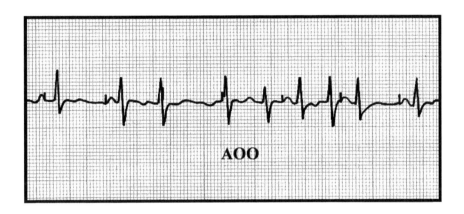

AOO

Functional noncapture results from pacing into native _____ _____.

Fusion with pacing is primarily a phenomenon of _____ pacing.

REFRACTORY PERIODS
VENTRICULAR

Chapter 12

DDD Pacing

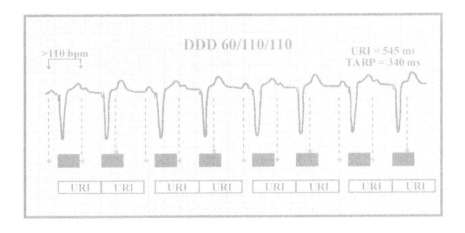

DDD PACING

DDD
↑
**PACES BOTH ATRIUM AND
VENTRICLE**

DDD
↑

**SENSES BOTH ATRIUM AND
VENTRICLE**

DDD
↑

**1) ATRIAL SENSING INHIBITS
ATRIAL PACING AND
TRIGGERS VENTRICULAR
PACING**

**2) VENTRICULAR SENSING
INHIBITS VENTRICULAR AND
ATRIAL PACING**

DDD PACING

In the early 1980s atrial sensing technology became incorporated into permanent dual-chamber pacemakers. From then implantation of DDD pacing systems steadily increased as physician confidence in reliable atrial lead function grew.

Today DDD pacing has become the dual-chamber pacing standard of care. While VVI pacing systems are still the most popular worldwide, DDD pacing systems encompass a greater percentage of the total number of new system implants in the United States, approximately 67% of new implants according to a 1993 survey of US physicians.

DDD pacing systems are more expensive and technically more challenging than VVI pacing systems, both to implant and to follow. On the upside, there exists substantial retrospective data demonstrating improved survival and decreased incidence of atrial fibrillation

(AF) with DDD versus VVI pacing. Ongoing prospective studies will shed further light on this issue.

Whatever the outcome of this issue, the ability of a pacemaker clinician to interpret and troubleshoot DDD pacing rhythms is paramount!

DDD Timing

Basic timing with DDD pacing includes three intervals, the lower rate interval (LRI), the atrioventricular or "AV" interval, and the ventriculoatrial or "VA" interval. Both the LRI and AV interval are programmed parameters, while the VA interval is not. The VA interval equals the LRI minus the AV interval or:

$$\textbf{LRI} = \textbf{VA} + \textbf{AV}$$

There is a slight variation to this rule with some types of pacemakers. More on this will follow shortly.

It cannot be stressed that knowing these three intervals is at the core of allowing a pacemaker clinician to understand most dual-chamber pacemaker ECGs!

The three basic timing intervals with DDD pacing include the programmed _____ and _____ interval, and the calculated _____ interval.

LRI, AV, VA

The AV interval is also known as the "ventricular escape interval." It is the period of time after a sensed or paced atrial event that the pacemaker will wait to see if an R wave occurs before pacing the ventricle.

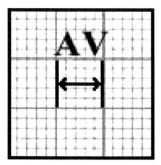

The AV interval is programmable. Typical programmed values are anywhere between 120 and 250 ms.

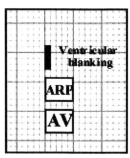

With the start of each AV interval the "atrial refractory period" (ARP) begins. This is a time during which no atrial event will be sensed and affect pacemaker timing. It is as long as the AV interval. Also at the start of the AV interval, *only after atrial pacing,* the "ventricular blanking period" begins. This is a short ventricular refractory interval (2040 ms) that serves to minimize the likelihood that an atrial pacing spike will be sensed as a ventricular event by the ventricular pacemaker channel.

Many pacemakers now allow two different AV intervals to be programmed, one to occur after P wave sensing (typically shorter), and the other to occur after atrial pacing (typically longer). Why?

The pacemaker starts the AV interval with P wave sensing after the P wave has already begun, and starts the AV interval with an atrial pacing spike before the P wave has really begun. Thus, two different AV intervals allow hemodynamic optimization of the time that the ventricular event happens after whatever atrial event precedes it.

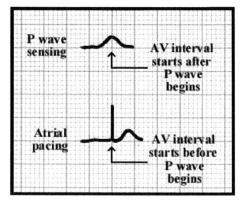

For the purposes of this book, only a single AV interval will be used from here on.

The AV interval is also known as the _____ _____ _____.

Ventricular blanking only occurs after _____ _____.

VENTRICULAR ESCAPE INTERVAL
ATRIAL PACING

A new AV interval begins each time that a sensed or paced atrial event occurs. The timing of each AV interval subsequently ends when either an R wave is sensed before the completion of timing, or when an R wave is not sensed resulting in ventricular pacing at the completion of timing.

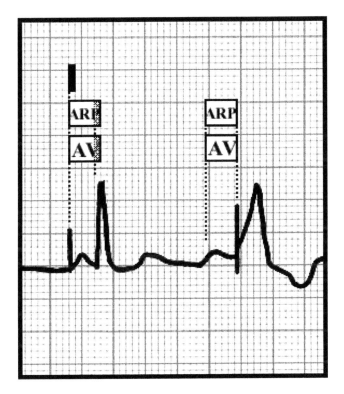

Helpful Hint: Measuring the AV interval backwards from a ventricular pacing spike will identify when atrial sensing occurred to initiate the interval.

A _____ or _____ atrial event will initiate a new AV interval with DDD pacing.

SENSED, PACED

The VA interval is also known as the "atrial escape interval." It is the period of time after a paced or sensed ventricular event that the pacemaker will wait to see if a P wave occurs before pacing the atrium.

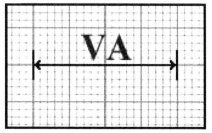

With the start of each VA interval, three other intervals also begin. The ventricular refractory period (VRP) serves to prevent the T wave from being sensed as a ventricular event. The postventricular atrial refractory period (PVARP; designated as ▇▇ on all ECGs that follow) serves to prevent a P wave occurring shortly after an R wave from being sensed. These refractory periods may be programmable and are usually on the order of 200 to 400 ms. No atrial events occurring during the PVARP or ventricular events during the VRP will affect pacemaker timing. The upper rate interval (URI) provides for a ceiling on how fast a dual-chamber pacemaker will allow the ventricle to be paced and is also programmable.

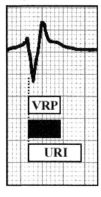

The VA interval is also known as the _____ _____ _____.

The _____ sets the ceiling on how fast the ventricle may be paced with a dual-chamber pacemaker.

ATRIAL ESCAPE INTERVAL
URI

A new VA interval begins each time that a sensed or paced ventricular event occurs (this includes a sensed premature ventricular contraction [PVC] during a VA interval!). The timing of each VA interval subsequently ends when either a P wave *or an R wave* (i.e., a PVC) is sensed before the completion of timing, or when neither a P wave or R wave is sensed resulting in atrial pacing at the completion of timing.

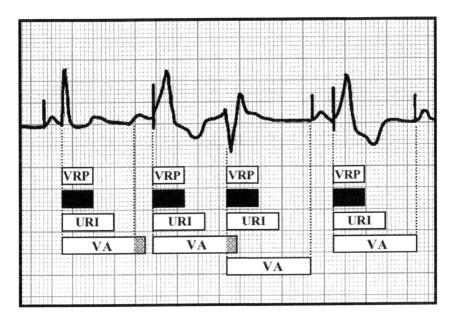

Helpful Hint: Measuring the VA interval backwards from an atrial pacing spike will identify when ventricular sensing occurred to initiate the interval.

A sensed or paced _____ event will initiate a new VA interval with DDD pacing.

VENTRICULAR

Putting it all together, a VA interval follows the timing for each AV interval and an AV interval follows the timing for each VA interval, except with a PVC that starts timing of a new VA interval.

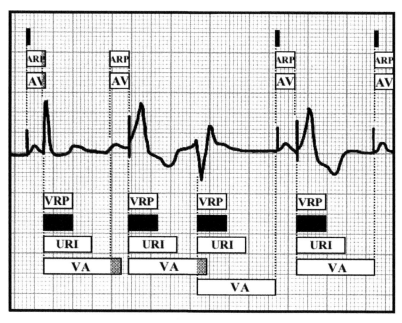

Encountering a short ECG rhythm strip as the one above that displays so many different combinations of atrial and ventricular pacing and sensing would be unusual. Patients with DDD pacing systems typically display a predominant rhythm that depends on how fast the native atrial rate is, and whether conduction down to the ventricle is intact or impaired. For example, if the predominant native atrial rate is faster than the lower rate, and ventricular conduction does not occur prior to the completion of each AV interval, a pattern of atrial sensing followed by ventricular pacing will predominate. What follows are more realistic patterns of pacing likely to be encountered.

The interval following each AV interval and sensed PVC is the _____ interval.

The interval following each VA interval, except with a sensed _____, is the _____ interval.

VA

PVC, AV

When the Atrial Rate is Less Than the Lower Rate and . . .

1) . . . there is no ventricular activity sensed during the AV interval

A pacemaker in the DDD mode will pace the atrium, and then the ventricle at the end of the AV interval, when the atrial rate is less than the lower rate, and there is no ventricular activity sensed in the AV interval. Timing of a new VA interval then begins after each ventricular paced event. The result is what is called "AV sequential" pacing at the lower rate.

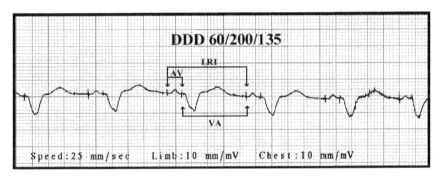

AV sequential pacing occurs when the ———— and then the ————, at the end of the AV interval, are paced.

In order for AV sequential pacing to occur when the lower rate is 60 pulses per minute (ppm) and the AV interval is 200 ms, the native rate must be ———— ———— ———— and the PR interval ———— ———— ————.

After a paced atrial event in the DDD mode a new ———— interval begins timing.

After a paced ventricular event in the DDD mode a new ———— interval begins timing.

ATRIUM, VENTRICLE
LESS THAN 60 bpm, GREATER THAN 200 ms
AV
VA

2) . . . there is sensed ventricular activity during the AV interval

A pacemaker in the DDD mode will pace the atrium and then sense the R wave, when the atrial rate is less than the lower rate, and the R wave occurs before the end of the AV interval. The sensed R wave inhibits ventricular pacing for that interval and starts the VA interval. The VA interval will equal the LRI minus the AV interval for what is called "ventricular based" pacing or somewhat longer than that with what is called "atrial based" pacing (see next page for explanations). There are two basic variations of atrial based pacing.

A sensed PVC occurring during the VA interval inhibits both atrial *and* ventricular pacing, and starts a new VA interval with ventricular based pacing and a most common form of atrial based pacing.

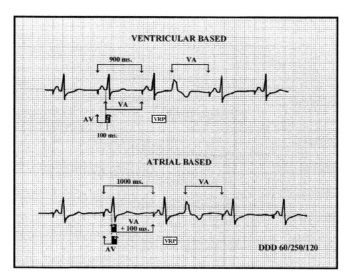

An R wave sensed during the AV interval (yet not too early so as to cause safety pacing) will _____ ventricular pacing for that interval.

Atrial and ventricular pacing are inhibited by _____ that occur after the VRP and during the VA interval with ventricular based pacing and a most common form of atrial based pacing.

INHIBIT
PVCs

Ventricular Versus Atrial Based Pacing, or "Pacing Base"

Pacing base determines how a dual-chamber pacemaker in the DDD, DDI, or DVI mode (more about DDI and DVI later) will respond to a sensed ventricular event during both the AV and VA intervals. It is nonprogrammable. The pacing base is determined by the preference of the pacemaker manufacturer and can be found by referring to the technical manual that comes with each new pacemaker.

Pacing base differences during the AV interval
(see previous page for illustration)

The effect of pacing base is evident when an R wave is sensed during the AV interval. With ventricular based pacing the atrium can be paced at a rate that is *faster* than lower rate, depending on how early in the AV interval each sensed R wave occurs. Atrial based pacing ensures that the atrium cannot be paced faster than the lower rate. For example, with ventricular based pacing, if each R wave occurs 100 ms before the end of the AV interval the atrium will be paced at an interval that is 100 ms shorter than the LRI. With atrial based pacing the VA interval is extended by 100 ms after the sensed R wave to ensure that the atrial pacing rate does not go above lower rate.

Pacing base differences during the VA interval
(see next page)

The effect of pacing base is evident during the VA interval when a PVC occurs. As mentioned on the previous page a sensed PVC during the VA interval inhibits both atrial *and* ventricular pacing and starts a new VA interval with ventricular based pacing and a most common form of atrial based pacing (sometimes called "modified atrial based" pacing). Another less common form of atrial based pacing ("pure atrial based" pacing) will sense a PVC during this interval, yet wait a time equal to the LRI before pacing the atrium. This attempts to mimic the compensatory pause that typically occurs after a PVC.

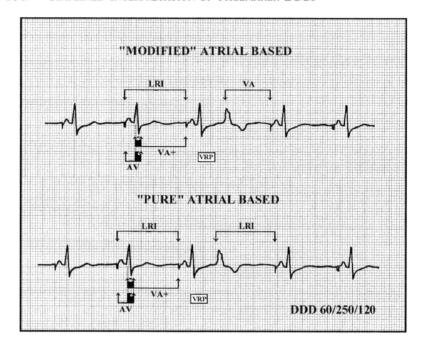

SAFETY PACING

Many dual-chamber pacemakers have a feature commonly referred to as "safety pacing." Safety pacing is a function that prevents ventricular pacing from being inappropriately inhibited by a noncardiac potential, i.e., pectoral muscle potential, or an atrial pacing spike, that is sensed by the ventricular lead during the AV interval. When a potential, cardiac or noncardiac, is sensed on the ventricular lead during the most early portion of the AV interval, an early ventricular pacing spike is triggered to occur. This protects patients with no native AV conduction, i.e., complete heart block, from having no stimulus for ventricular activation.

Safety pacing is often a sign of loss of atrial sensing. Here's how: When P waves are not sensed the VA interval can often complete timing and pace the atrium just before or during the first portion of the native R wave that follows the non-sensed P wave. The R wave is then sensed early in the AV interval and triggers a safety pacing spike.

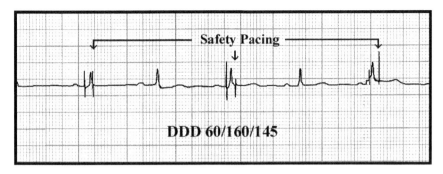

Noncardiac potentials or an atrial pacing spike sensed early in the AV interval may trigger a _____ _____.

Safety pacing can often be a sign of loss of _____ _____.

SAFETY PACE
ATRIAL SENSING

CROSSTALK

It may rarely happen that the atrial pacing output is sufficiently large such that it is sensed as a ventricular event by the ventricular channel immediately after the ventricular blanking period. This process is called "crosstalk." Decreasing the atrial pacing output and/or decreasing the ventricular sensitivity can generally avoid crosstalk. In some pacemakers the ventricular blanking period may also be programmed longer.

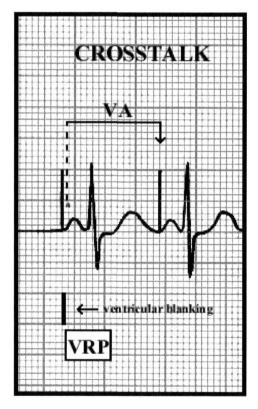

The name of the process that occurs when an atrial pacing output is sensed by the ventricular channel is _____.

CROSSTALK

Crosstalk can be lethal in patients with no native ventricular escape and no safety pacing! It may be suspected when there is no ventricular pacing output at the end of an AV interval without an R wave occurring in it, following an atrial pacing output. Persistent safety pacing following atrial pacing should also raise the suspicion of crosstalk. Crosstalk with ventricular based pacing results in a shortened atrial pacing interval (A-A) while with atrial based pacing the A-A interval is maintained at the LRI.

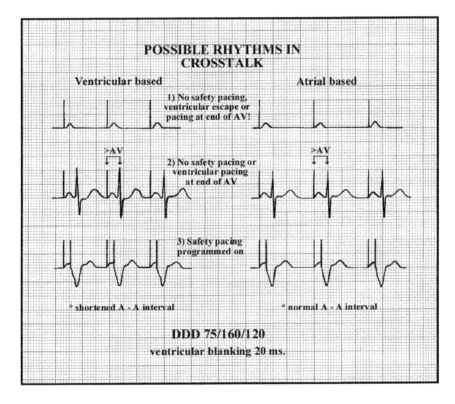

Persistent safety pacing following atrial pacing should raise the suspicion of _____.

The absence of safety pacing and a native ventricular escape can be _____ during crosstalk.

CROSSTALK
LETHAL

When the Atrial Rate is Greater Than the Lower Rate and . . .

1) . . . there is sensed ventricular activity during the AV interval

A pacemaker in the DDD mode will sense both P waves occurring after the PVARP and the subsequently conducted R waves when the atrial rate is greater than lower rate and the R waves occur before the end of the AV interval. Each sensed P wave inhibits atrial pacing and initiates the AV interval while each sensed R wave inhibits ventricular pacing for that cycle. The response to the sensed R wave depends on the pacing base.

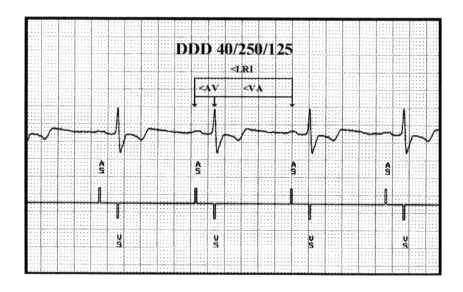

In the DDD mode, P waves are sensed when occurring after the _____ and before the VA interval ends, will _____ atrial pacing for each cycle that they are sensed, and will initiate the ____ interval.

PVARP, INHIBIT, AV

Intact atrial sensing cannot be confirmed by analyzing the surface ECG when the AV interval is greater than the PR interval and the VA interval is greater than the interval between successive R waves ("R-R" interval). The surface ECG will look identical whether atrial sensing is present or not. Here's how:

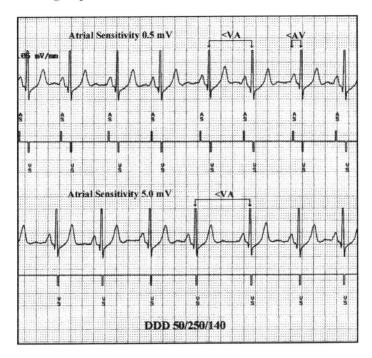

With intact atrial sensing atrial pacing is inhibited by each P wave sensed after the PVARP. The AV interval is then initiated. Since the PR interval is less than the AV interval, ventricular pacing is inhibited by each sensed R wave. No pacing outputs are seen.

With absent atrial sensing each R wave is sensed prior to completion of the preceding VA interval. Each time this occurs atrial *and* ventricular pacing are inhibited since the R wave is interpreted by the pacemaker as a PVC. No AV intervals are initiated. Again no pacing outputs are seen.

The presence of atrial sensing is not known by looking at the surface ECG when the AV interval is _____ than the PR interval and the VA interval is _____ than the R-R interval.

GREATER, GREATER

2) ... there is no sensed ventricular activity during the AV interval

A pacemaker in the DDD mode will sense each P wave occurring after the PVARP and trigger pacing in the ventricle at the end of the AV interval, when the atrial rate is greater than the lower, *but* less than the upper rate, and there is no sensed ventricular activity during the AV interval. This pacing sequence is also commonly called "P wave tracking" or "atrial synchronous ventricular pacing."

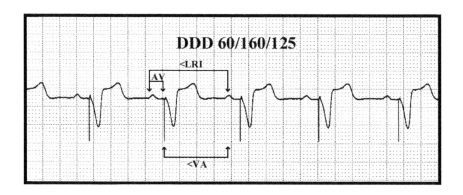

In the DDD mode, if P waves occur above the pacemaker lower rate, but less than the upper rate, and there is no sensed ventricular activity during the AV interval, the pacemaker will _____ the P waves and _____ the ventricle at the end of the AV interval.

This sequence of pacing is also called _____ _____ _____
or _____ _____ _____ _____.

SENSE, PACE
P WAVE TRACKING, ATRIAL SYNCHRONOUS VENTRICULAR PACING

Upper Rate Behavior

With faster P wave tracking, near or above the upper rate limit, interesting things start to happen!!!

Two types of P wave tracking behavior can be seen when P waves begin occurring close to or above the upper rate limit. What will be seen depends on how the pacemaker has been programmed.

When the URI is greater than the total atrial refractory period (PVARP + AV interval, or "TARP") pacemaker Mobitz type I block or "Wenckebach" block will be seen as P waves occur at a rate greater than the upper rate limit. Here's why:

Since P waves occurring faster than the upper rate can still be sensed before they fall into the PVARP, the AV interval will progressively lengthen so as to not pace the ventricle faster than the upper rate limit. Eventually a P wave will fall into the PVARP and not be sensed. The sequence then repeats itself.

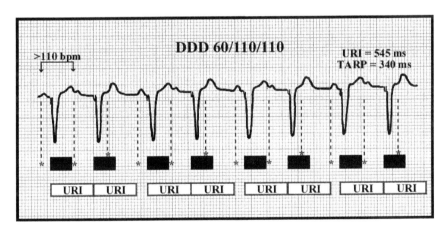

Mobitz type I block upper rate P wave tracking occurs when the _____ is greater than the _____ _____ _____ _____.

Mobitz type I block is also known as _____ block.

URI, TOTAL ATRIAL REFRACTORY PERIOD (PAVRP + AV IN-TERVAL)
WENCKEBACH

The second type of P wave tracking upper rate behavior occurs when the URI is less than or equal to the TARP. As P waves go faster one will fall into the PVARP and not be sensed, before or at the same time that upper rate limit is reached. This results in "dropped beats" or Mobitz type II block (no prolongation of the AV interval). Typically the block is 2:1 (two P waves for every ventricular paced beat).

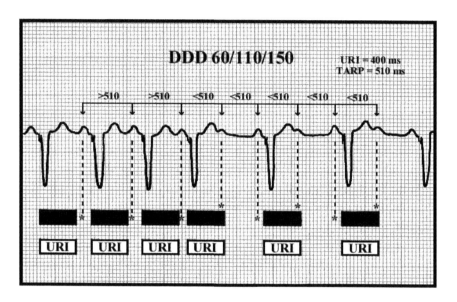

The TARP equals the _____ interval plus the _____.

Mobitz type II block upper rate P wave tracking occurs when the URI is _____ than the TARP.

With Mobitz type II block the AV interval _____ _____ prolong.

AV, PVARP
LESS
DOES NOT

PACEMAKER-MEDIATED TACHYCARDIA

Ventricular pacing can cause conduction backwards in a patient's heart that activates the atria. This is called "retrograde atrial activation" and results in a "retrograde P wave." If the P wave occurs after the PVARP it can be sensed and trigger ventricular pacing at the end of the AV interval. The process can then continually repeat itself. This is called "pacemaker-mediated tachycardia" (PMT). When it occurs the ventricle is typically paced at the upper rate limit. PMT can be aborted by removing atrial sensing (easily done by placing a magnet on the pacemaker). Programming the PVARP longer such that each retrograde P wave falls into it, and thus is not sensed, will cure PMT.

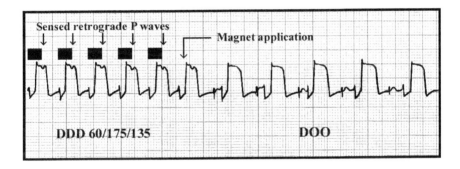

Continuous   sensing   of   a   retrograde   P   waves   results in _____ _____ _____.

Placement of a _____ on pacemaker will abort an episode of PMT.

PACEMAKER MEDIATED TACHYCARDIA
MAGNET

An important point to consider when the ventricle is being persistently paced at the upper rate limit, and there are no identifiable P waves, is that the pacemaker may be tracking AF. Upper tracking occurs because the AF waves are frequently sensed immediately after the end of the PVARP.

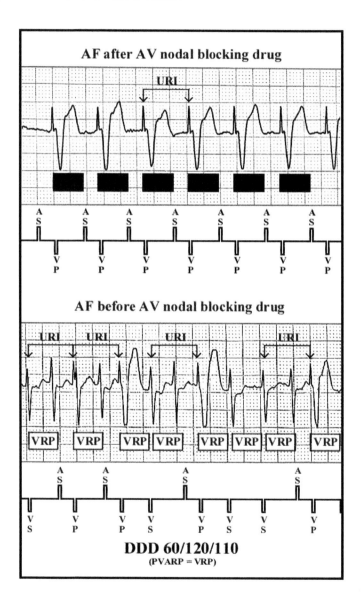

When AF is rapidly conducted via the native conduction system ventricular pacing spikes may appear to occur too close to the preceding R wave. Measuring the URI backwards from the ventricular pacing spikes is helpful in identifying what ventricular events were sensed to begin the URI. Superimposing the VRPs from these events is useful for demonstrating which subsequent R waves fall into the refractory period and are non-sensed. Thus, when these non-sensed R waves are taken into account it is seen that the ventricular pacing spikes all occur at upper rate and not too fast.

Tracking of _____ is a common cause of persistent DDD mode ventricular pacing at the upper rate limit.

AF

MODE SWITCHING

Many dual-chamber pacemakers have a programmable feature called "mode switching" which, when turned on, can identify when the heart rhythm has become AF, or for that matter any fast supraventricular tachycardia, and automatically change the pacemaker to a mode of pacing that will not track the atrium to the upper rate limit (VVIR, VDIR, DDIR). If sinus rhythm returns, mode switching will recognize this and return the pacemaker to the initial pacing mode.

In order for mode switching to function the pacemaker needs to be able to recognize when rapid atrial rhythms are occurring, even during refractory periods!

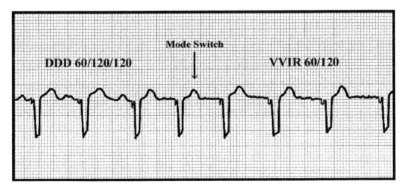

AF can be recognized by a pacemaker with _____ _____ and automatically change the mode to one that will not track AF.

MODE SWITCHING

RATE MODULATION

Rate modulation in the DDDR mode will progressively increase the atrial pacing rate with exertion. If the AV interval is greater than the PR interval then ventricular pacing will be inhibited with each cycle, and only atrial pacing will be seen. This rhythm will appear exactly the same as if an AAIR pacing mode was in effect (For those of you keeping track, this rhythm strip *is* the same one used earlier to demonstrate AAIR pacing, as well as a DDIR and DVIR rhythm strip to come later.)

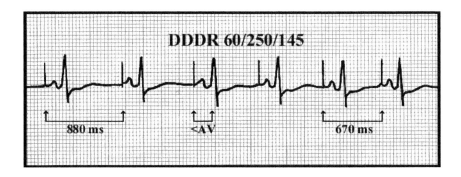

A simple way to tell whether the pacing mode with atrial pacing only seen on ECG is AAIR versus one of DDDR/DDIR/DVIR is to place a _____ on the pacemaker.

MAGNET

As rate modulation increases the pacing rate in the DDDR mode the AV interval may progressively shorten in order to optimize cardiac hemodynamics. This is a feature that is usually programmable ("ON" versus "OFF") and will obviously only be evident on the surface ECG when the AV intervals are less than the PR interval. The process of changing AV interval with pacing rate is sometimes called "AV interval hysteresis."

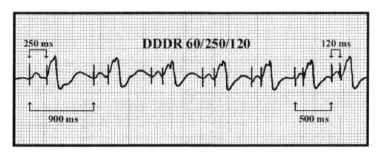

Changing of the _____ interval with increasing pacing rate in the DDDR mode is sometimes called _____ _____.

AV, AV INTERVAL HYSTERESIS

With rate modulation there may be competition between the P wave rate and the sensor-indicated atrial pacing rate such that the ECG rhythm displays both P wave tracking and atrial pacing.

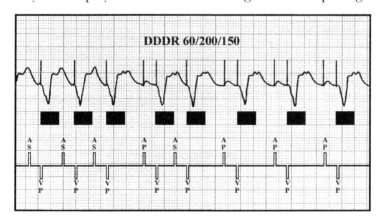

P wave tracking and sensor-indicated atrial pacing may _____ during exertion.

COMPETE

Magnet Mode (DOO)

Placement of a magnet on a DDD(R) pacemaker will cause it to pace both chambers asynchronously at the magnet rate regardless of the underlying rhythm. *It does not sense* (got the idea yet?)! If the native rhythm is slower than the magnet rate then atrial and ventricular capture will most likely be seen at the magnet rate.

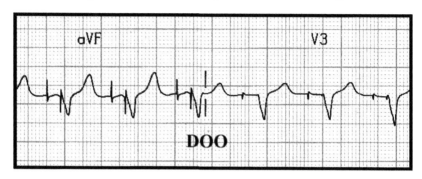

_____ pacing occurs when a magnet is placed on a pacemaker in the DDD(R) mode.

With a DOO pacing mode there is no _____.

DOO
SENSING

When the native rhythm is faster than the magnet rate periods of atrial and ventricular capture, functional noncapture, and ventricular fusion may be seen.

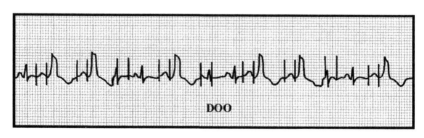

Functional noncapture occurs when pacing into na- tive _____ _____.

REFRACTORY PERIODS

Chapter 13

VDD Pacing

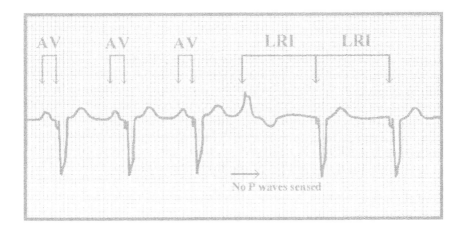

VDD PACING

VDD
↑
PACES THE VENTRICLE ONLY

VDD
↑
**SENSES BOTH ATRIUM AND
VENTRICLE**

VDD
↑

**1) ATRIAL SENSING
TRIGGERS VENTRICULAR
PACING**

**2) VENTRICULAR SENSING
INHIBITS VENTRICULAR PACING**

VDD PACING

The VDD mode is a pacing mode that is rarely seen. Its functions are the same as the DDD mode, except that it does not pace the atrium. Thus it loses its application of atrioventricular (AV) synchrony (P wave tracking) in the frequently encountered patient whose indication for pacing is sinus bradycardia. Another way of thinking of this is that the VDD mode functions as a VVI pacemaker that can also track P waves.

A niche that the VDD mode has attempted to fill is with the use of a single pacemaker lead that can perform all ventricular functions, yet also sense P waves. Engineers have designed a pacemaker lead whose tip inserts into the right ventricle (RV) to pace and sense, and with electrodes in its body that float freely in the atrium and sense P waves. Unfortunately, the freely floating electrodes may not 100% reliably sense the P waves.

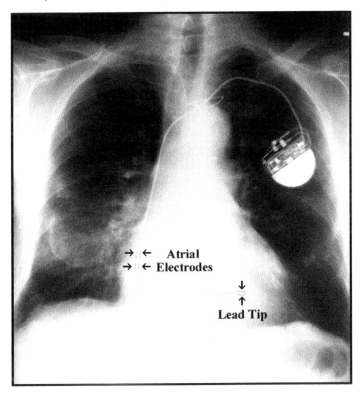

There is no ⎯⎯⎯⎯ ⎯⎯⎯⎯ in the VDD mode.

P waves may be _____ in the VDD mode.

ATRIAL PACING
SENSED

VDD TIMING

The basic timing intervals of importance for VDD pacing include the AV interval and the lower rate interval (LRI). Calculation of the ventriculoatrial (VA) interval is generally not helpful because there is no atrial pacing that can occur at its conclusion.

The AV interval with VDD pacing is the time after a sensed P wave that the pacemaker will wait to see if an R wave occurs before pacing the ventricle. It is programmable. An atrial refractory period (ARP) is also initiated with the onset of P wave sensing and lasts as long as the AV interval is timed. There is no ventricular blanking period initiated because there is no atrial pacing.

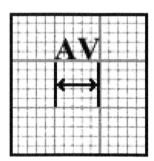
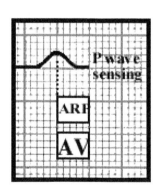

P wave sensing with VDD pacing initiates an ___ interval, an ___, but not a _____ _____ ___.

Calculating the VA interval with VDD pacing is generally not useful because there is no _____ _____.

AV, ARP, VENTRICULAR BLANKING PERIOD
ATRIAL PACING

A new AV interval begins each time that a sensed P wave occurs. The timing of each AV interval subsequently ends when either an R wave is sensed before the completion of timing or when an R wave is not sensed resulting in ventricular pacing at the completion of timing.

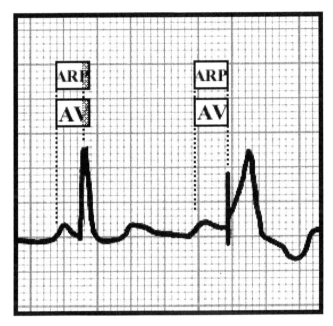

Only a _____ atrial event initiates an AV interval with VDD pacing.

SENSED

The LRI is the period of time after a paced or sensed ventricular event that a VDD pacemaker will wait to see if either a P or R wave occurs before pacing the ventricle.

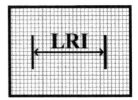

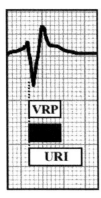

With the initiation of each LRI three other intervals also begin. They are the ventricular refractory period (VRP), postventricular atrial refractory period (PVARP), and the upper rate interval (URI). Their functions serve exactly the same purpose as that for a DDD pacing mode. No atrial events occurring within the PVARP or ventricular events occurring within the VRP will affect pacemaker timing.

During the LRI after the refractory periods, a VDD pacemaker is alert to sense either a _____ or _____.

A P wave occurring during the PVARP _____ _____ be sensed and affect pacemaker timing.

P WAVE, R WAVE
WILL NOT

A new LRI begins each time that a sensed or paced ventricular event occurs. The timing of each LRI subsequently ends when P wave triggered ventricular pacing occurs before the completion of timing, an R wave is sensed before the completion of timing, or no R wave is sensed before completion of timing resulting in ventricular pacing at the end of timing.

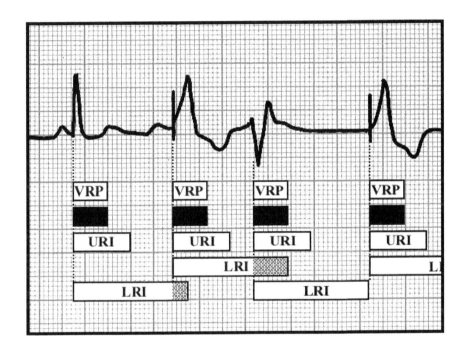

A _____ or _____ ventricular event starts the timing of a new LRI in the VDD mode.

SENSED, PACED

Putting it all together a new LRI follows the timing of each preceding LRI. (Sounds a lot like a single-chamber pacemaker!) When a sensed P wave occurs an AV interval is triggered within.

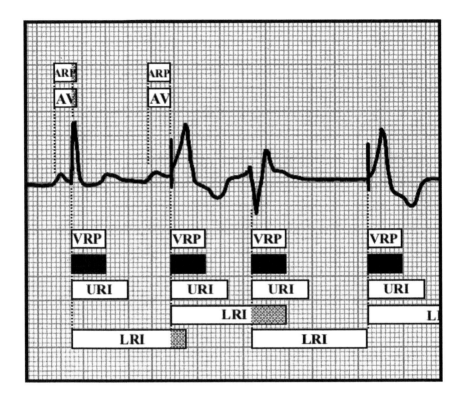

With VDD pacing a new _____ follows each preceding LRI.

LRI

When the Atrial Rate is Greater Than the Lower Rate and . . .

1) . . . there is sensed ventricular activity during the AV interval

A pacemaker in the VDD mode will behave exactly as if it were in the DDD mode for rhythms that completely inhibit pacing (native rate > lower rate, R wave sensed during each AV interval).

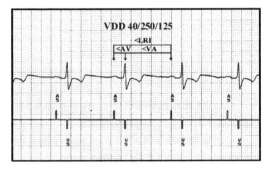

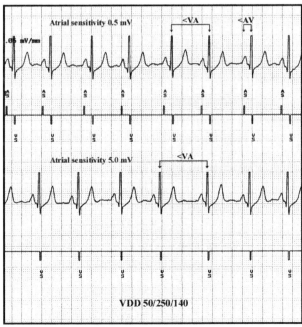

Atrial sensing cannot be confirmed by looking at the surface ECG when the R-R interval is _____ than the VA interval, and the PR interval is _____ than the AV interval.

LESS, LESS

2) . . . there is no sensed ventricular activity during the AV interval

As in the DDD mode, sensed P waves will trigger ventricular pacing at the end of the AV interval in the VDD mode. This occurs so long as there is no sensed ventricular activity during the AV interval.

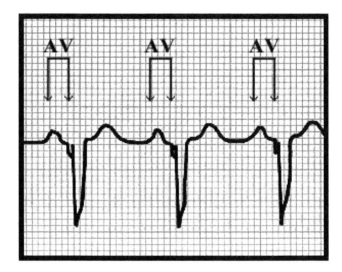

The VDD mode shares a function of the DDD mode in that it will _____ ventricular pacing at the end of an AV interval devoid of sensed ventricular activity.

TRIGGER

When P Waves are Not Sensed

When there is no sensed atrial activity, the VDD mode function-ally becomes VVI (senses R waves and paces the ventricle at the LRI when needed). Another way of thinking of this is that the VDD mode is a VVI pacemaker with the ability to track P waves.

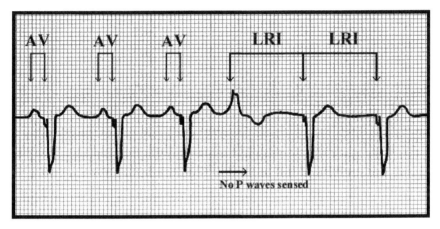

A pacemaker programmed to the VDD mode will act as if pro-grammed to the _____ mode until there is sensed atrial activity.

VVI

When P Waves Occur Just Before the LRI Finishes

If P waves occur after the VA interval ends, but before the LRI finishes, they will be sensed, start an AV interval, and result in ventricular pacing at the end of the AV interval (assuming there is no sensed ventricular activity during the AV interval). The resultant ventricular paced interval is slightly greater than the LRI.

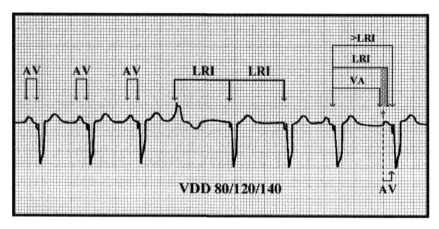

A ventricular paced interval slightly greater than the LRI can occur in the VDD mode when a P wave is sensed after the _____ interval and before completion of the _____.

VA, LRI

VDD Upper Rate Behavior

A VDD pacing mode will behave exactly the same as in the DDD mode to P wave tracking rhythms at the upper rate.

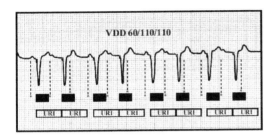

Mobitz I Block

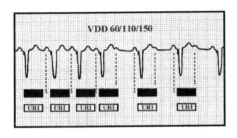

Mobitz II Block

and . . .

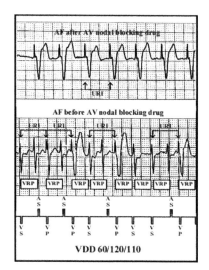

Atrial Fibrillation

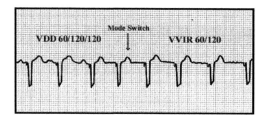

Mode Switching

Upper rate tracking behavior in the VDD mode is exactly the same as in the _____ mode.

DDD

Magnet Mode (VOO)

Magnet mode for VDD pacing is VOO. How fast the native rhythm is will determine what is seen on the surface ECG (ventricular capture versus a combination of ventricular capture, fusion, and functional noncapture).

Slow native rhythm

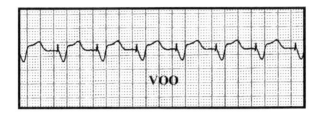

Fast native rhythm

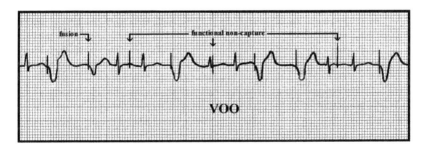

VOO is the magnet mode for both _____ and _____ pacing modes.

VVI, VDD

Chapter 14

DDI Pacing

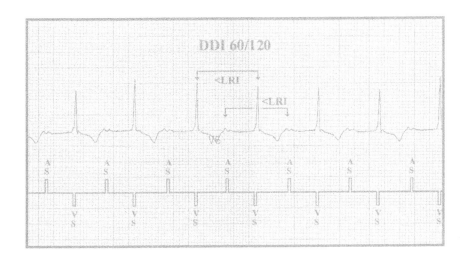

DDI PACING

DDI
↑
**PACES BOTH ATRIUM AND
VENTRICLE**

DDI
↑
**SENSES BOTH ATRIUM AND
VENTRICLE**

DDI
↑
**1) ATRIAL SENSING INHIBITS
ATRIAL PACING AND DOES
NOT TRIGGER VENTRICULAR
PACING**

**2) VENTRICULAR SENSING
INHIBITS VENTRICULAR AND
ATRIAL PACING**

DDI PACING

This mode is the one frequently found to be the most difficult to understand (it was for me too!). The confusion stems from the fact that: 1) it is an infrequently used mode of pacing, and 2) atrial pacing will initiate an atrioventricular (AV) interval while a sensed atrial event will inhibit atrial pacing, but *will not* initiate an AV interval. Therefore, P wave tracking cannot occur. This is not so good for maintaining AV synchrony in the presence of heart block. In fact, the only way AV synchrony is maintained with this mode is if complete inhibition of pacing with normal native AV conduction occurs or the atrial rate is less than the lower rate. If the point of using dual-chamber pacing is to maintain AV synchrony, then why use this mode of pacing at all?

Initially, it was typically used to AV sequentially pace patients with paroxysmal atrial fibrillation (AF), and avoid sudden pacing at the upper rate limit from tracking of the AF waves. Automatic mode switching in the DDD mode resolved that issue.

The DDIR mode in devices without mode switching can be found somewhat more useful than DDI for maintaining AV synchrony. It will allow an increased atrial pacing rate (remember atrial pacing initiates an AV interval) and not track paroxysmal AF.

P wave tracking _____ occur in the DDI mode.

In the DDI mode, paced atrial events _____ and sensed atrial events _____ _____ initiate an AV interval.

CANNOT
DO, DO NOT

DDI Timing

Basic timing with DDI pacing includes the AV interval, the ventriculoatrial (VA) interval, and the lower rate interval (LRI).

The AV interval with DDI pacing is the time after atrial pacing that the pacemaker will wait to see if an R wave occurs before pacing the ventricle.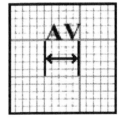

With the start of each AV interval the atrial refractory period (ARP) begins. This is a time during which no atrial event will be sensed and 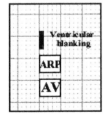 affect pacemaker timing. It is as long as the AV interval. Also at the start of the AV interval the ventricular blanking period begins. This period serves to minimize the likelihood that an atrial pacing spike will be sensed as a ventricular event by the ventricular pacemaker channel.

The _____ interval is also known as the ventricular escape interval.

The ventricular blanking period decreases the likelihood that an _____ _____ _____ is sensed by the ventricular channel.

AV
ATRIAL PACING SPIKE

A new AV interval begins each time that atrial pacing occurs. The timing of each AV interval subsequently ends when either an R wave is sensed before the completion of timing or when an R wave is not sensed resulting in ventricular pacing at the completion of timing.

A new ARP begins each time that an atrial event, paced *or* sensed, occurs. After a sensed P wave it lasts until the next ventricular event.

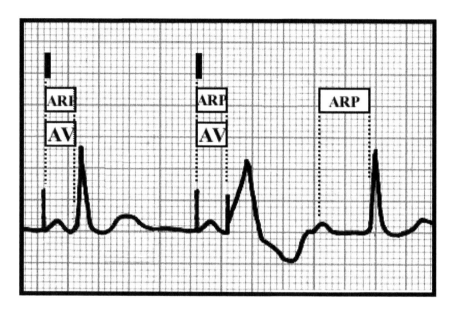

In the DDI mode an AV interval is initiated only with _____ _____.

A paced or sensed atrial event initiates an _____ in the DDI mode.

ATRIAL PACING
ARP

The VA interval is the period of time after a paced or sensed ventricular event that the pacemaker will wait to see if a P wave occurs before pacing the atrium.

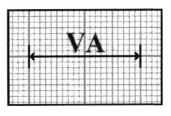

With the start of each VA interval two other intervals also begin. The ventricular refractory period (VRP) serves

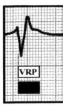

to prevent the T wave from being sensed as a ventricular event. The postventricular atrial refractory period (PVARP) serves to prevent a P wave occurring shortly after an R wave from being sensed. No atrial events occurring during the PVARP or ventricular events during the VRP will affect pacemaker timing. There is no upper rate interval (except for DDIR pacing) since there is no P wave tracking.

The _____ interval is also known as the atrial escape interval.

VA

A new VA interval begins each time that a sensed or paced ventricular event occurs. The timing of each VA interval subsequently ends when either a P wave or an R wave is sensed before the completion of timing, or when neither is sensed resulting in atrial pacing at the completion of timing.

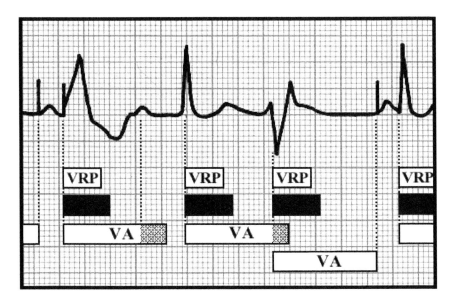

A _____ or _____ ventricular event will initiate a new VA interval with DDI pacing.

SENSED, PACED

Since atrial sensing does not initiate an AV interval, the LRI serves as the interval that the pacemaker will wait before pacing the ventricle when atrial sensing occurs during it.

A new LRI follows each sensed or paced ventricular event. Each LRI subsequently finishes timing when either an R wave is sensed before the completion of timing, or when an R wave is not sensed resulting in ventricular pacing at the completion of timing.

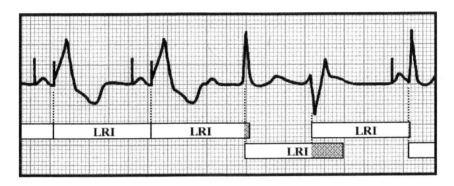

In the DDI mode a _____ event initiates and ends each LRI.

The point of possible ventricular pacing after a sensed P wave is determined by the _____ that started before it.

VENTRICULAR
LRI

Putting it all together, a new LRI follows the timing of each preceding LRI. The timing of an AV interval occurs within this period only following a completed VA interval (i.e., when no atrial sensing occurs).

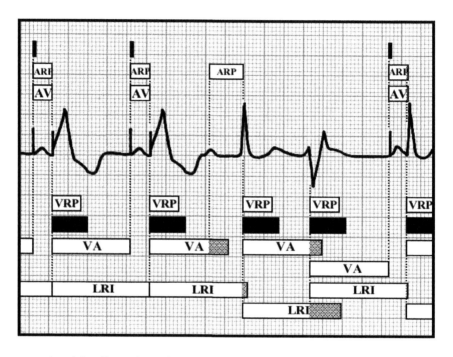

As with all modes of pacing, a predominant pacing pattern can usually be identified based on how fast the native atrial rate is with respect to the lower rate and whether AV conduction occurs before the AV interval completes timing. Some examples of this now follow.

An AV interval follows a _____ VA interval.

COMPLETED

When the Atrial Rate is Less Than the Lower Rate and . . .

1) . . . there is no sensed ventricular activity during the AV interval

First the atrium, and then the ventricle will be paced in the DDI mode when the atrial rate is slower than the lower rate and there are no R waves sensed during the AV interval.

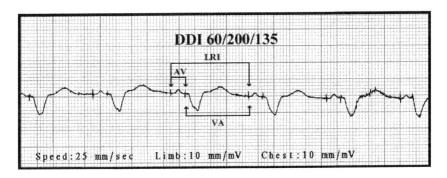

The pattern of atrial pacing followed each time by ventricular pacing is called _____ pacing.

In order for AV sequential pacing to occur when the native atrial rate is 50 bpm and the PR interval is 200 ms, the lower rate of pacing must be _____ _____ _____ and the AV interval _____ _____ _____.

AV SEQUENTIAL
GREATER THAN 50 bpm, LESS THAN 200 ms

2) . . . there is sensed ventricular activity during the AV interval

A pattern of atrial pacing will be seen on the surface ECG when the native atrial rate is less than the lower rate and R waves are sensed prior to completion of each AV interval. How the pacemaker reacts to the R wave sensed during the AV interval is determined by the pacing base. (Remember this? If not, check out the DDD pacing section again! The example below displays "modified" atrial based pacing.)

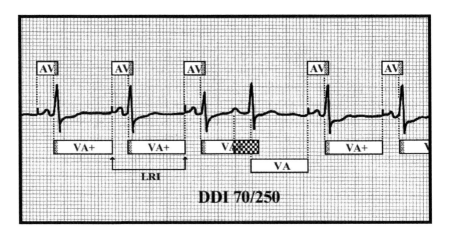

If the rate that the atrium is paced in the DDI mode, with atrial pacing followed by ventricular sensing for each cycle, is maintained at the lower rate, then the pacing base must be _____ based.

In the DDI mode an AV interval is only started following an atrial _____ event, and not after an atrial _____ event.

ATRIAL
PACED, SENSED

When the Atrial Rate is Greater Than the Lower Rate and . . .

1) . . . the ventricular rate is greater than the lower rate

Complete inhibition of pacing in the DDI mode can occur when the native atrial and ventricular rates are greater than the lower rate. Again, P waves are sensed in the DDI mode, but *do not* initiate an AV interval.

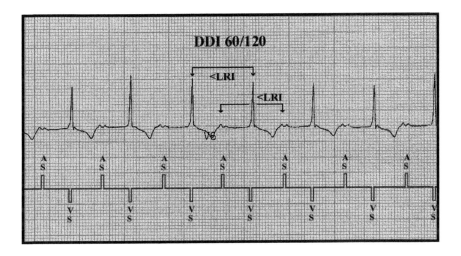

Multiple other rhythms with atrial and ventricular rates greater than the lower rate are possible, and depend on how the pacemaker is programmed, what the pacing base is, and whether there is a high degree of heart block. (These possibilities are too numerous, and become too confusing for this basic text so will not be covered.)

P wave tracking *does not* occur in the _____ mode.

DDI

When the R-R interval is less than the VA interval atrial sensing cannot be confirmed by analyzing the surface ECG alone in the DDI mode no matter what the PR interval (so long as the P waves are outside the PVARP). The surface ECG will look the same whether or not atrial sensing is intact. Here's why:

Atrial Sensitivity 0.5 mV

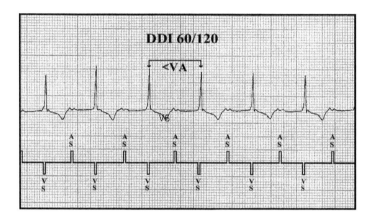

Atrial Sensitivity 5.0 mV

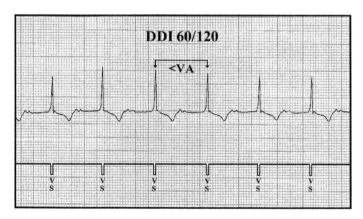

With intact atrial sensing atrial pacing is inhibited by each P wave sensed after the PVARP. No AV interval is initiated. Each subsequent R wave inhibits ventricular pacing. Thus no pacing outputs occur.

With absent atrial sensing each subsequent R wave is sensed prior to completion of the VA interval. Each time this occurs atrial and ventricular pacing are inhibited. Again no pacing outputs occur.

The presence of atrial sensing is not known by looking at the surface ECG when the _____ interval is less than the _____ interval.

R-R, VA

2) . . . the ventricular rate is less than the lower rate

P waves will be sensed until one falls into the PVARP when the atrial rate is greater than the lower rate and the ventricular rate is less than the lower rate. Ventricular pacing *does not* occur any faster than the lower rate in the DDI mode (except if in the DDIR mode).

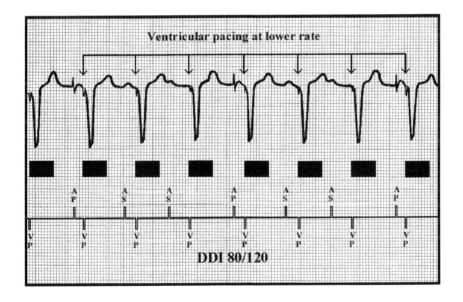

Ventricular pacing can only occur at the _____ _____ in the DDI mode.

LOWER RATE

Since there is no triggering of ventricular pacing by sensed atrial activity in the DDI mode, the sudden onset of AF (i.e., paroxysmal AF) poses no problem. The pacemaker just paces the ventricle at the LRI when there is no native ventricular activity.

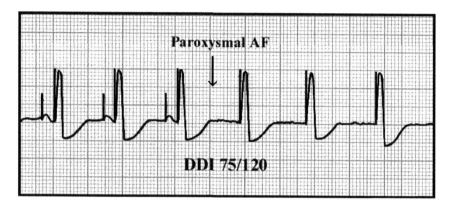

A DDI pacemaker will pace the ventricle at the LRI when there is _____ atrial activity and no native ventricular activity.

SENSED

RATE MODULATION

Rate modulation in the DDIR will increase the atrial pacing rate with exertion in the absence of sensed atrial activity. If R waves are sensed during the AV interval, ventricular pacing will be inhibited and only atrial pacing will be seen. If no R waves are sensed during the AV interval then AV sequential pacing will occur. As the atrial pacing rate increases the AV interval can be programmed to shorten to optimize cardiac hemodynamics.

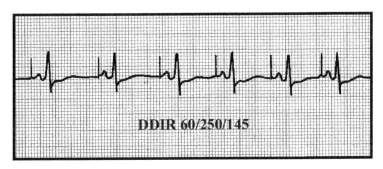

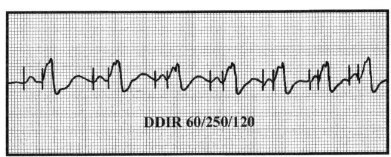

Atrial pacing rate will _____ with exertion in the DDIR mode.

INCREASE

Should the native atrial rate be faster than the sensor indicated atrial pacing rate in the DDIR mode, the P waves will be sensed until one falls into the PVARP. The giveaway that rate modulation is in effect with this type of rhythm is to note the change in *ventricular* pacing interval (remember that in plain DDI pacing the ventricular pacing interval is fixed at the LRI).

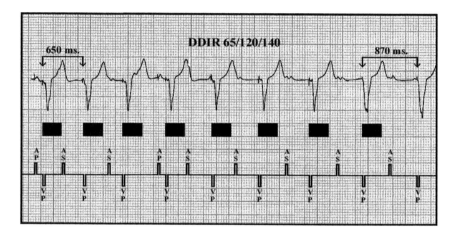

The _____ pacing interval is not fixed at the LRI in the DDIR mode.

VENTRICULAR

Magnet Mode (DOO)

Magnet mode for a DDI(R) pacemaker is DOO. Pacing will occur asynchronously in both chambers, regardless of the underlying rhythm, at the magnet rate. If the native rhythm is slower than the magnet rate then AV sequential capture at the magnet rate will occur. With a native rhythm faster than the magnet rate a combination of atrial and ventricular capture, functional noncapture, and ventricular fusion may happen.

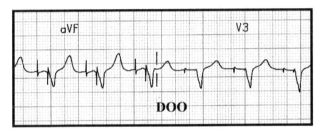

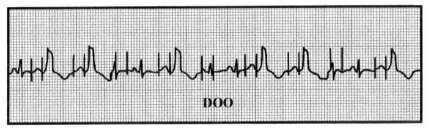

With the DOO mode there is no _____ or _____ sensing.

ATRIAL, VENTRICULAR

Chapter 15

DVI Pacing

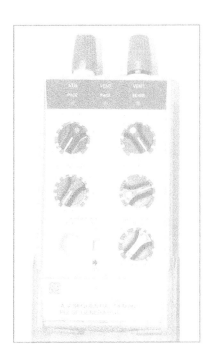

DVI PACING

DVI
↑
**PACES BOTH ATRIUM AND
VENTRICLE**

DVI
↑
**SENSES THE VENTRICLE
ONLY**

DVI
↑
**VENTRICULAR SENSING
INHIBITS ATRIAL AND
VENTRICULAR PACING**

DVI Pacing

This was the first permanent dual-chamber pacing mode. Time has since rendered it fairly obsolete, as reliable atrial sensing with

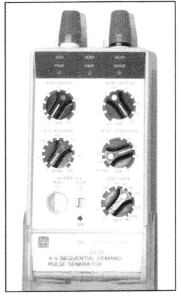

DDD pacing has become the permanent dual-chamber pacing standard of care. So why mention it? Many external dual chamber-pacing boxes without atrial sensing (i.e., DVI pacing) are still utilized. They can frequently be found as temporary external pacing devices. Therefore it is helpful to know its function. Also, if atrial sensing in a DDD mode fails, the resultant functional pacing mode becomes DVI until such time that loss of atrial sensing is remedied.

Of note, some of the examples that follow do not display safety pacing with early ventricular sensing in the atrioventricular (AV) interval. Temporary external pacing boxes (save the newest models) and the earliest permanent versions of DVI pacing typically do not have this function.

Of note, some of the examples that follow do not display safety pacing with early ventricular sensing in the atrioventricular (AV) interval. Temporary external pacing boxes (save the newest models) and the earliest permanent versions of DVI pacing typically do not have this function.

With DVI pacing there is no atrial _____.

DVI pacing is frequently used as a _____ external pacing device.

SENSING
TEMPORARY

DVI TIMING

Basic timing with DVI pacing includes the AV interval, the ventriculoatrial (VA) interval, and the lower rate interval (LRI).

The AV interval with DVI pacing is the time after atrial pacing that the pacemaker will wait to see if an R wave occurs before pacing the ventricle.

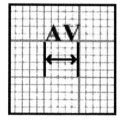

With the start of each AV interval the ventricular blanking period begins. This period serves to minimize the likelihood that an atrial pacing spike will be sensed as a ventricular event by the ventricular pacemaker channel.

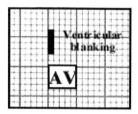

Since there is no atrial sensing with the DVI mode, no AV intervals are initiated with a P wave. Another way of thinking of this is that the atrial pacemaker channel is always in refractory.

An AV interval begins only with _____ _____ in the DVI mode.

ATRIAL PACING

A new AV interval begins each time that atrial pacing occurs. The timing of each AV interval subsequently ends when either an R wave is sensed before the completion of timing or when an R wave is not sensed resulting in ventricular pacing at the completion of timing.

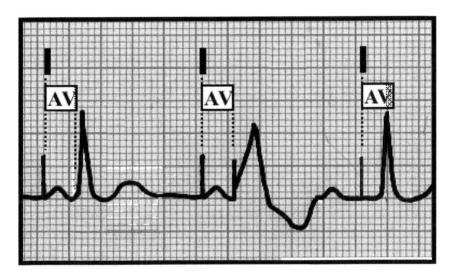

In the DVI mode an _____ interval is initiated only with atrial pacing.

AV

The VA interval is the time after a paced or sensed ventricular event that the pacemaker will wait before pacing the atrium.

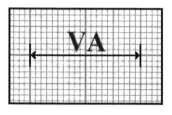

With the start of each VA interval only a ventricular refractory period (VRP) is initiated. Since there is no P

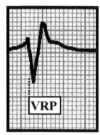

wave sensing there is no postventricular refractory period (PVARP) and no upper rate interval (URI) (except with DVIR pacing).

A new VA interval begins each time that a sensed or paced ventricular event occurs. The timing of each VA interval subsequently ends when either an R wave is sensed before the completion of timing, or one is not sensed resulting in atrial pacing at the completion of timing.

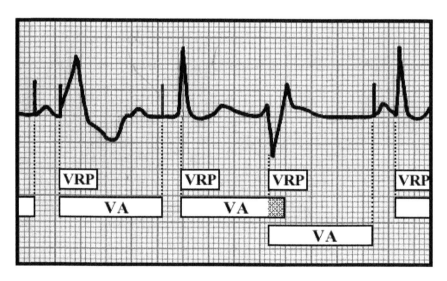

A _____ is, and a _____ or _____ are not initiated with each VA interval.

VRP, PVARP, URI

Putting it all together, a VA interval follows the timing for each AV interval and an AV interval follows the timing for each VA interval, except with an R wave sensed during the VA interval that starts timing of a new VA interval.

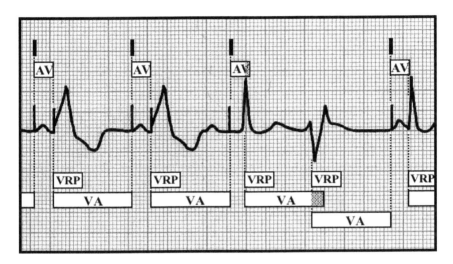

Now onto more examples likely to be found in clinical practice!

When an R wave is sensed during a VA interval in the DVI mode _____ and _____ pacing are inhibited and a new _____ interval is initiated.

ATRIAL, VENTRICULAR, VA

When the Atrial Rate is Less Than the Lower Rate and . . .

1) . . . no ventricular activity occurs during the AV interval

AV sequential pacing and capture will occur with the DVI mode when the native atrial rate is less than the lower rate and no R waves are sensed during the AV interval. Atrial capture may not functionally happen if a P wave occurs faster and just prior to an atrial pacing spike. If a premature ventricular contraction is sensed, it will inhibit atrial and ventricular pacing and start a new VA interval.

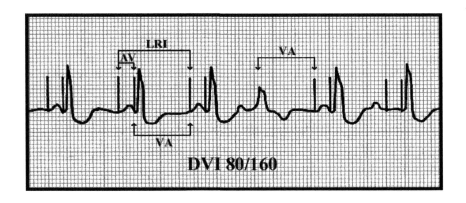

Functional atrial non-capture can occur with a P wave that happens just _____ an atrial pacing spike.

BEFORE

2) ... ventricular activity is sensed during the AV interval

Atrial pacing will occur in the DVI mode when the native atrial rate is less than the lower rate and R waves are sensed during the AV interval (modified atrial based pacing seen below).

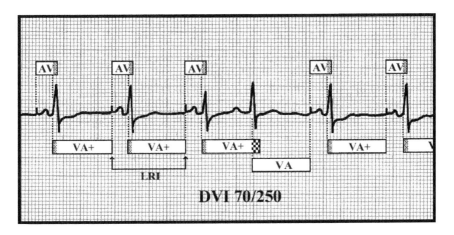

DVI 70/250

For example, if the lower rate is 70 pulses per minute (ppm), and the AV interval is 250 ms, in order to see atrial pacing only on the ECG in the DVI mode the native atrial rate must be _____ _____ and the PR interval _____ _____ 250 ms.

LESS THAN 70 bpm, LESS THAN

When the VENTRICULAR Rate is Greater Than the Lower Rate and . . .

1) . . . the R-R interval is less than the VA interval

Complete pacemaker inhibition will occur when the ventricular rate is greater than the lower rate and the R-R interval is less than the VA interval. This happens because each R wave is sensed prior to the end of each VA interval, and thus inhibits both atrial and ventricular pacing each cycle.

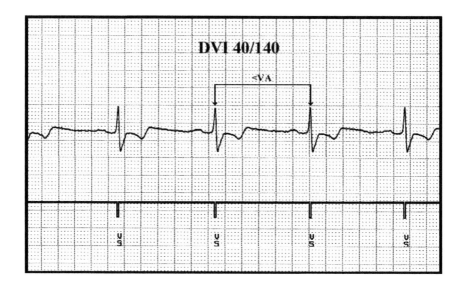

In order for complete pacing inhibition to occur in the DVI mode, the _____ rate must be greater than the lower rate, and the _____ interval less than the VA interval.

VENTRICULAR, R-R

2) . . . the R-R interval is slightly greater than the VA interval

An atrial pacing spike will occur just prior to the R wave when the R-R interval is slightly greater than the VA interval. Ventricular based pacing and no safety pacing are evident in the example below.

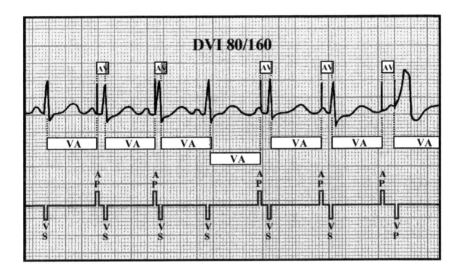

In the DVI mode, atrial pacing spikes can normally occur in the PR interval because there is no _____ _____.

R waves sensed during the VA interval in the DVI mode will _____ both _____ and _____ pacing.

ATRIAL SENSING
INHIBIT, ATRIAL, VENTRICULAR

Because there is no atrial sensing in the DVI mode, atrial spikes can often occur during a native PR interval. The subsequent R wave that occurs early in the AV interval will trigger safety pacing if the device has this property.

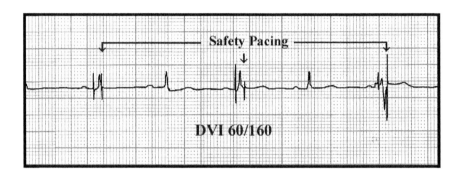

_____ _____ is a dual-chamber pacemaker function that prevents ventricular pacing from being inappropriately inhibited by a non-cardiac potential or atrial pacing spike sensed early in the AV interval.

The presence of safety pacing often signifies lack of _____ _____.

SAFETY PACING
ATRIAL SENSING

RATE MODULATION

As in the other dual-chamber pacing modes, rate modulation in the DVIR mode will increase the atrial pacing rate, if needed, with exertion. Whether or not an R wave is sensed during the AV interval will determine what pattern of pacing is seen, atrial or AV sequential.

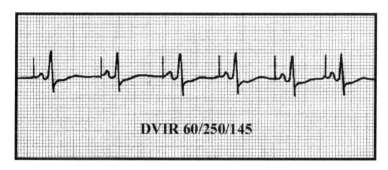

DVIR 60/250/145

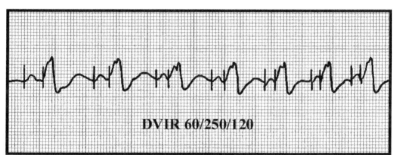

DVIR 60/250/120

Either _____ or _____ pacing can be seen with DVIR pacing.

ATRIAL, AV SEQUENTIAL

Magnet Mode (DOO)

Magnet mode for DVI(R) pacing is DOO. As in the other dual-chamber modes with atrial and ventricular pacing, the pacing pattern seen on the ECG depends on whether the native rate is faster or slower than the magnet rate.

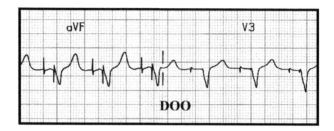

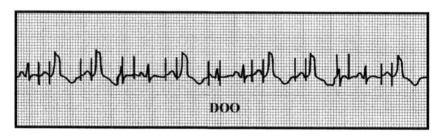

Section III

Unusual Pacing Situations and Alternate Applications of Permanent Pacing

Chapter 16

Unusual Pacing Situations

Pre-AMI treatment

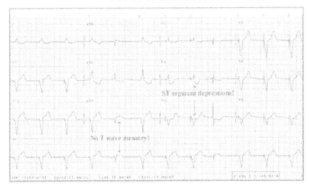

Post-AMI treatment

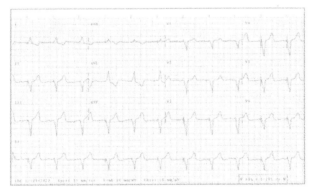

Diagnostic Pacing Modes

There are pacemaker modes that are useful for their diagnostic properties when evaluating a patient's pacing system. It should be stressed, however, that only experienced individuals should use them. The reason will become evident shortly.

OAO – senses atrium
OVO – senses ventricle
ODO – senses atrium & ventricle

None of these modes have pacing capabilities, and as such are not recommended in patients who are pacemaker dependent unless used as a "temporary" mode by an experienced individual. Temporary modes are modes available with the use of a pacemaker programmer that can be turned off in a split second with reversion to the permanent pacemaker programmed mode. Their use comes into play when wanting to assess for an underlying rhythm. Marker channels can also be run in these modes purely to assess sensing capabilities.

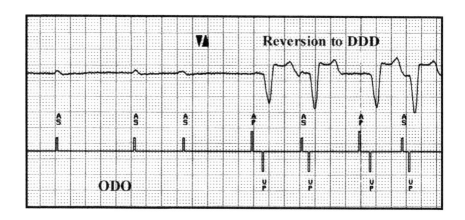

Use of pacing modes without active pacing function are recommended in _____ circumstances and only by _____ individuals.

TEMPORARY, EXPERIENCED

The following modes can also be used to help evaluate sensing, but are essentially outdated and no longer used.

AAT – senses atrium which triggers pacing in atrium
VVT – senses ventricle which triggers pacing in ventricle

These modes use pacing spikes as markers to identify when sensing has occurred. The spikes do not capture.

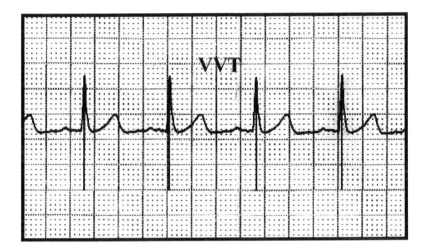

Again, diagnostic pacing modes are primarily useful for evaluating pacemaker _____ under _____ circumstances.

SENSING, TEMPORARY

PACING TO PREVENT ATRIAL FIBRILLATION

Current research is under way investigating the use of atrial pacing as a means of preventing atrial fibrillation (AF). It is widely felt that atrial pacing may create an electrical environment in atrial cardiac tissue that is less likely to sustain AF, and will also prevent premature atrial contractions (PACs) that may lead to the initiation of AF. As such some pacemakers now have pacing algorithms designed to maintain atrial pacing as much of the time as possible. Frequently having the pacemaker automatically lower its rate until the native atrial rate is found and then adjusting atrial pacing to a slightly faster rate is one such algorithm. Also having the pacemaker adjust the atrial pacing rate upwards after detecting a PAC is another.

Some investigators are also examining whether simultaneous atrial pacing from multiple sites can prevent AF. It remains to be seen, however, to what degree such treatments may have on preventing AF. Currently, permanent pacing is not indicated solely for the purpose of prevention of AF.

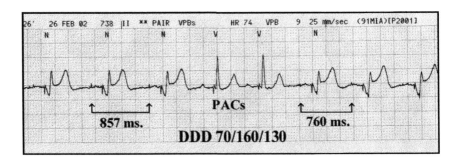

Current research is being conducted for the use of _____ pacing for the prevention of AF.

Maintaining atrial pacing at a rate _____ than the native atrial rate may help create an environment less favorable for sustaining AF.

ATRIAL
FASTER

Transcutaneous Pacing

Before the introduction of transvenous pacing wires a man by the name of Paul Zoll developed external pacing "pads," often called "Zoll pads," that can be used to pace the heart. The pads are placed on the front and back of the chest, and attached to an external pacing device. When turned on, the heart can be paced. In addition though, the skeletal muscles of the chest can contract with each pacing pulsation causing a generous amount of discomfort to the patient.

In clinical application today they are used mainly for emergency pacing purposes. It is often impossible to tell from the surface ECG whether the heart is actually being captured as the large amount of energy needed to externally stimulate the heart obliterates the surface signal. Thus, it is important to palpate the patient's pulse and measure the patient's blood pressure to confirm effective pacing capture.

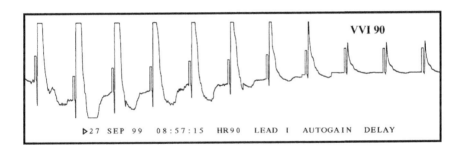

External pacing pads are often referred to as _____ _____.

The surface ECG is often _____ due to the large amount of energy required to externally pace the heart.

ZOLL PADS
OBLITERATED

AUTOMATIC THRESHOLD DETERMINATION

Certain types of pacemakers are able to automatically determine ventricular pacing threshold! This is typically done numerous times over the course of each day. Once the threshold is found the pacemaker adjusts the ventricular pacing output to be just above the threshold. This function serves to maximize battery life by minimizing the amount of energy needed for each ventricular pacing pulse.

During the threshold test in one such device, the pacemaker adjusts the pacing output downward until it detects that it has not captured the heart. The pacemaker then adjusts the pacing output upward to define the threshold. Each time that the pacemaker detects noncapture during the test, a suprathreshold "rescue pacing spike" is delivered shortly after the subthreshold testing spike to ensure uninterrupted capture.

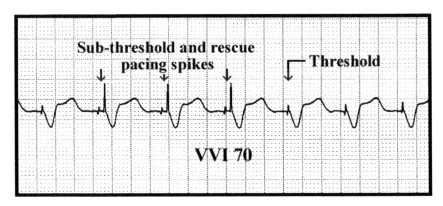

Pacing capture threshold is defined when the pacing energy is adjusted _____ after losing capture.

Automatic threshold determination is used to _____ the amount of energy used by the pacemaker for ventricular pacing.

UPWARDS
MINIMIZE

DIAGNOSIS OF MYOCARDIAL INFARCTION

It is difficult, if not impossible, to make the diagnosis of acute myocardial infarction (AMI) from an ECG during ventricular pacing. This is because the typical ECG findings of AMI, ST segment elevation, may not be seen during ventricular pacing. This should not preclude obtaining a 12-lead ECG during ventricular pacing when a patient has the signs and symptoms consistent with an AMI, as there are ECG changes suggestive of it. This includes the presence of ST segment depression, or ST segment elevation of ≥5 mm in ECG leads where the paced QRS is predominantly negative. In ECG leads where the paced QRS is positive, ST segment elevation has also been found to be a specific sign of AMI. It cannot be stressed enough, however: *The absence or presence of such ECG findings during ventricular pacing should not stop or delay the treatment for AMI if the history and physical exam are consistent with it!*

Temporary inhibition of ventricular pacing to examine the native QRS complexes for ST segment changes can be done, but is not always practical, and may not show the typical findings during AMI due to a phenomenon called "T wave memory." T wave memory is a process that can occur following the cessation of ventricular pacing and can cause an alteration of the ST segment and T wave that masks the typical ECG findings one might see during AMI.

ECG findings during ventricular pacing suggestive of AMI include ST segment _____, or _____ _____ in ECG leads where the QRS is predominantly negative.

The absence or presence of ECG changes consistent with AMI during ventricular pacing _____ _____ alter the management of a patient suspected of having an AMI.

Following the cessation of ventricular pacing, the typical ECG findings during AMI may not be seen due to a phenomenon called _____ _____.

DEPRESSION, ELEVATION ≥5 mm
SHOULD NOT
T WAVE MEMORY

Pre-AMI treatment

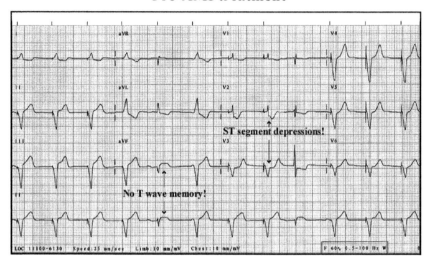

Post-AMI treatment

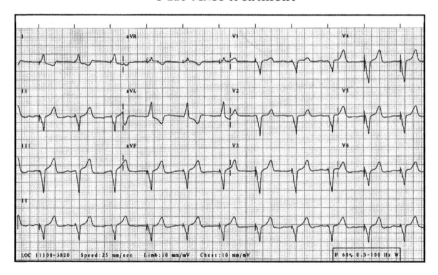

Effects of Electric Cautery on Pacing

The use of electric cautery ("bovi") in the operating room can have profound effects on a permanent pacing system. First, it obscures interpretation of the surface ECG (the simultaneous use of pressure waveform monitoring is helpful in this regard to assure the presence of a heartbeat). Second, the signal from the electric cautery can be sensed by the pacemaker and inappropriately inhibit pacing. Finally, a pacemaker whose battery is at end of life can suddenly fail when exposed to the cautery signal. This would not be good for someone who is pacemaker dependent. Thus, it is especially important to consider a back-up pacing measure (i.e., a temporary transvenous pacing wire) to prevent the potential tragic consequences of such an occurrence.

Electric cautery is also referred to as a _____.

Electric cautery can obscure the _____, inappropriately _____ pacing, and cause a battery at end of life to suddenly _____.

BOVI
ECG, INHIBIT, FAIL

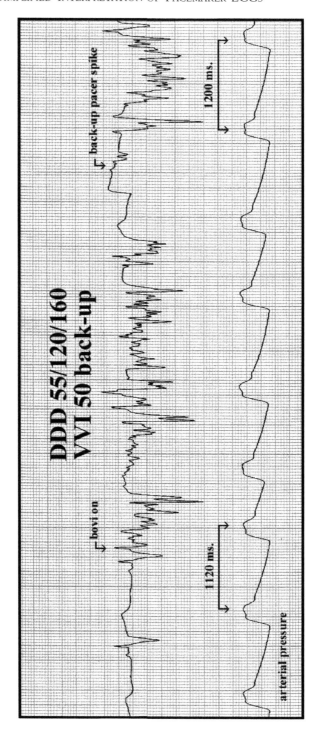

Chapter 17

Alternate Applications of Permanent Pacing

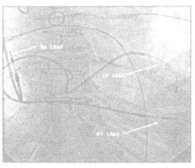

Pacing for Hypertrophic Obstructive Cardiomyopathy

Hypertrophic obstructive cardiomyopathy (HOCM) is a type of abnormal heart muscle growth characterized by left and/or right ventricular hypertrophy and a thickening of the septum between the left and right ventricle (LV, RV) that impedes the exit of blood from the LV. This may cause significant symptoms including chest pain, lightheadedness, or syncope. Quite often it is diagnosed with an echocardiogram.

One type of treatment, after the use of certain medications, is the use of a dual-chamber pacemaker. Here's how it works:

The normal electrical activation of the thickened ventricular septum causes it to contract in a manner such that it may further obstruct blood flow from the LV. By pacing the RV, the left side of the septum is electrically activated to contract later. This, along with an increased delivery of blood volume to the LV from a synchronous atrial contribution, may actually widen the opening for blood flow from the LV. There is current controversy, however, as to whether this type of treatment actually provides any symptomatic benefit.

HOCM may result in the _____ of blood flow from the LV.

Pacing the RV may actually _____ the opening for blood flow from the LV.

OBSTRUCTION
WIDEN

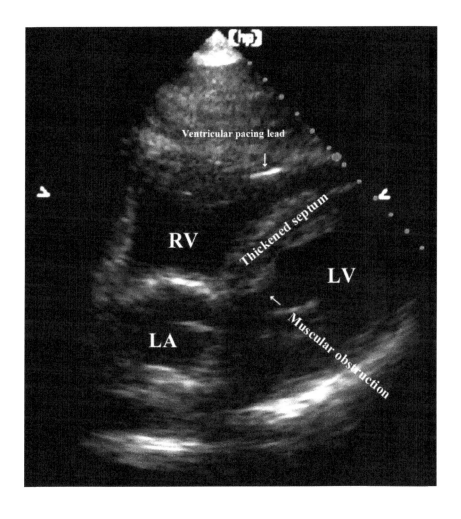

PACING FOR VENTRICULAR TACHYCARDIA

Implantable cardioverter-defibrillators (ICDs) are devices that treat tachyarrhythmias, in particular ventricular tachycardia (VT) and ventricular fibrillation (VF). The initial treatment modality after detecting VT can be programmed to something called "overdrive or burst pacing."* Overdrive pacing is a short burst of ventricular pacing at a rate that is slightly faster than the VT. The sudden cessation of this can result in the VT being terminated. Overdrive pacing cannot be used to terminate VF.

The newer generations of ICDs also have pacemaker capabilities. This becomes helpful in two respects: 1) many patients are on drugs to treat VT, which may significantly slow the baseline heart rate, and 2) many times after treatment and termination of VT or VF there can be a significant pause or period of bradycardia. Pacemaker functions of ICDs can be tailored to treat both cases.

VT can be treated by ICDs with _____ or _____ pacing.

VF _____ be treated by overdrive pacing.

ICDs also have _____ functions, which can treat pauses or brady-cardia.

BURST, OVERDRIVE
CANNOT
PACEMAKER

---

*This form of pacing may also be referred to as "anti-tachycardia" pacing. Older generations of pacemakers included such function, and were used for treating atrial tachyarrhythmias. Now, they do not include anti-tachycardia pacing.

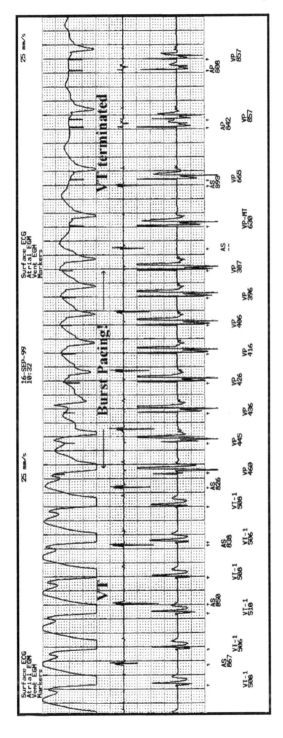

Pacing for Heart Failure

One of the more recent applications of permanent pacing has been for the treatment of severe heart failure. This came about because many patients whose hearts have poor pumping function also have abnormal electrical activation of the heart muscle. This can typically manifest as first-degree atrioventricular block and/or bundle branch block. These problems are not traditional indications for permanent pacing. When these delays occur the heart muscle does not contract in a normal fashion.

Studies have shown that a more "normal" electrical activation of the heart muscle in these patients may improve cardiac performance, and thereby improve heart failure symptoms.

For this to happen separate leads are implanted to pace the right *and* left ventricle (i.e., bi-ventricular pacing). The left ventricular lead is inserted into a coronary sinus vein (a vein that drains into the right atrium), or placed on the surface of the LV by performing a left thoracotomy. A right atrial lead is also implanted. A special pacemaker or defibrillator attached to this system is programmed to pace/sense the atria, and then pace both ventricles in a synchronized fashion. The more "normal" ventricular activation may result in a narrower QRS complex on the surface ECG. Study results of this type of treatment have led the Food and Drug Administration to recently approve bi-ventricular pacing for specific patients with heart failure.

Pacing/sensing the atrium and then both right and ___ ventricles attempts to normalize the electrical activation sequence in heart failure patients with bundle branch block.

LEFT

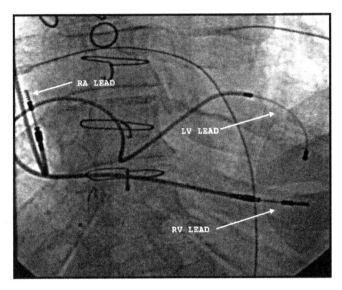

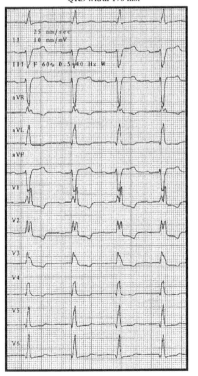

Baseline
QRS width 170 ms.

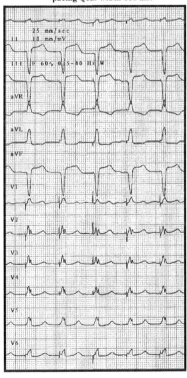

Bi-ventricular
pacing QRS width 110 ms.

Pacing for Syncope

Permanent pacing has also been investigated as a treatment for a specific type of syncope that involves rapid drops in heart rate within the normal range of heart rates and below. Investigators are trying to determine if providing an elevated paced heart rate, when this drop begins to occur, can prevent this type of syncope. The patient often does not use permanent pacing other than in these instances. Hence the lower rate is typically programmed low. Here's how it all works:

The pacemaker used for this treatment is able to detect drops in the patient's own heart rate within a specified short period of time. The clinician is able to specify what heart rate drop and in what period of time that it happens will trigger the treatment. When the drop occurs the pacemaker will respond with a faster pacing rate,* again predetermined by the clinician, in hopes of catching the process early and aborting it. It remains to be seen whether this treatment will prove to be beneficial.

Syncope can occur with a rapid drop in ＿＿＿＿＿ ＿＿＿＿＿.

Pacing for the treatment of syncope involves detecting the episode ＿＿＿＿＿ in an attempt to ＿＿＿＿＿ it.

HEART RATE
EARLY, ABORT

---

*This manner of pacing response is a form of hysteresis that may be referred to as "negative" hysteresis; a hysteresis interval that is shorter than the programmed lower rate interval.

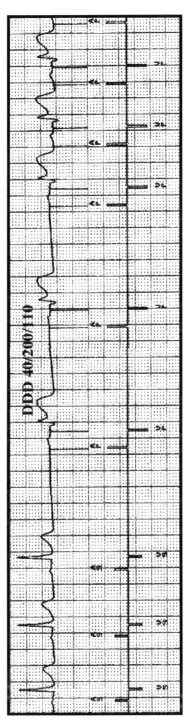

Section IV

Case Studies

Much more often than not an evaluation to "rule out pacemaker malfunction" shows the system to be working appropriately and the ECG reading to be incorrect. It is the rarer circumstance where there is a malfunction that needs to be recognized. "Pacemaker malfunction" is a misnomer as malfunctions almost never occur with the pacemaker generator itself, but rather occur somewhere within the pacemaker lead or its interface with the heart.

What follows are exercises to aid the "rule out pacemaker malfunction" process.

Chapter 18

Case Studies Part A

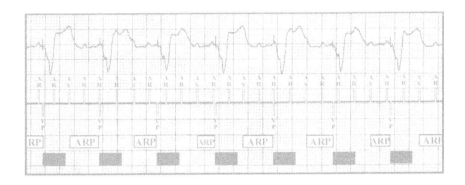

CASE STUDIES PART A

Quite often, analysis of a pacemaker ECG is undertaken without an available pacemaker programmer or any knowledge of the programmed parameters. A useful exercise for enhancing the ability to interpret pacemaker ECGs for these instances is to determine as much information as possible from the ECG without resorting to the use of a programmer even when one is available. Of particular interest are the mode, lower rate interval (LRI) and atrioventricular (AV) and ventriculo-atrial (VA) intervals (for dual-chamber pacemakers).

In this part the mode and parameters are not given. Determining the possible mode(s) of pacing is the goal of each exercise. Function is *normal* for each of these cases. Many times multiple different modes of pacing can produce the same pacemaker rhythm. This should be fairly evident by now from Section II. Identification of atrial, ventricular, or both types of pacing spikes and as many of the LRI, AV, and VA intervals helps narrow this process.

These cases, as well as those in Part B of this section, are given a rating that appears after each case number ( ). As the number of stars increases, so does the difficulty of interpreting each ECG.

✳	**Easiest**
✳✳	**Harder**
✳✳✳	**Moderately Difficult**
✳✳✳✳	**Very Difficult**
✳✳✳✳✳	**Most Difficult**

CASE 1 (✷)

What mode(s) of pacing could produce this rhythm? (Assume ventricular based pacing for dual-chamber modes.)

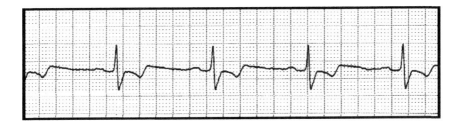

VVI, AAI, DDI, DVI, VDD, DDD

Complete pacing inhibition occurs on this strip. Therefore no asynchronous modes (AOO, VOO, DOO) are possible. AAI and VVI pacing modes with the native rate greater than the lower rate can completely inhibit pacing.

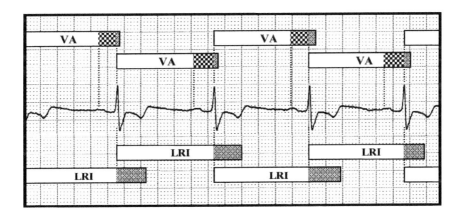

This rhythm will also completely inhibit pacing with a DDI mode when each P wave occurs before the end of each VA interval and the R-R interval is less than the LRI. Pacing can be completely inhibited with DVI pacing when the R-R interval is less than the VA interval. This occurs as each sensed R wave inhibits both atrial and ventricular pacing with each cycle.

Finally, VDD or DDD pacing with a lower rate less than the native rate, *and* an AV interval greater than the PR interval will completely inhibit pacing. This occurs because each VA and AV interval ends before completion of timing with a sensed P and R wave, respectively.

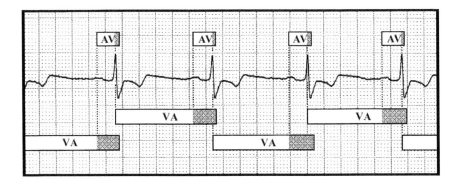

CASE 2 (✷)

What mode(s) of pacing could produce this rhythm?

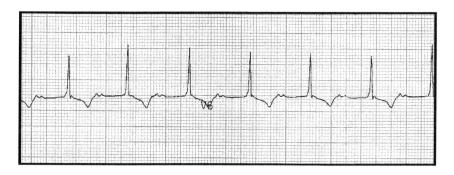

VVI, DVI, or DDI

As in the previous case there is complete pacing inhibition, so the AOO, VOO, and DOO pacing modes are not possible. AAI and VVI pacing with the native rate greater than the lower rate will completely inhibit pacing. However, given the severe first-degree AV block it is unlikely an AAI system was initially implanted. There is no P wave tracking, so the VDD and DDD modes would not produce this rhythm. This rhythm will also completely inhibit pacing with a DDI mode when each sensed P wave occurs before the end of each VA interval and the R-R interval is less than the LRI, and with DVI pacing when the R-R interval is less than the VA interval. This occurs with the DVI mode as each sensed R wave inhibits both atrial and ventricular pacing with each cycle.

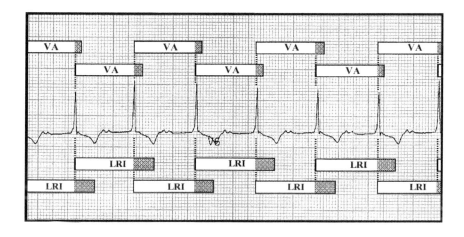

CASE 3 (✽)

What pacing mode(s) could produce this rhythm?

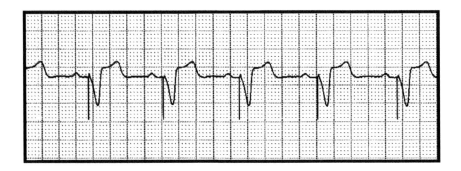

VDD or DDD

The ventricular pacing spikes all appear to occur at the same time after each P wave, suggesting P wave tracking. DDD and VDD pacing can obviously accomplish this while the other modes cannot.

P waves can rarely occur isorhythmically with ventricular pacing (i.e., same rate) such that the appearance of P wave tracking can be mimicked. Over a very short period of time, however the lack of AV synchrony becomes obvious as respiration alters the P wave rate while the ventricular pacing rate remains fixed.

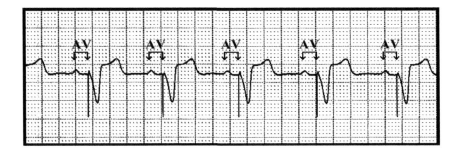

CASE 4 (✳✳✳)

What mode(s) of pacing could produce this rhythm?

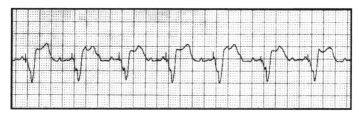

VVI, VOO

The ventricular pacing is obvious and bears no relationship to the rapid underlying atrial activity (atrial flutter), i.e., it is not tracked. There are no atrial pacing spikes. That removes DOO and DVI pacing. Because there are no native R waves, both VVI and VOO pacing are still possible.

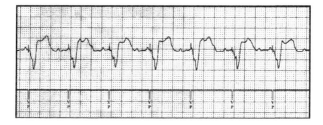

or . . .

DDI, DDD/VDD with mode switching

Complete atrial pacing inhibition from the atrial flutter,* with ventricular pacing at the LRI, makes DDI pacing possible. Mode switching from the atrial flutter in the DDD and VDD modes with resultant VVI pacing could also occur.

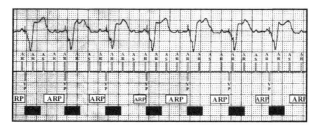

*Some pacemaker marker channels also note when events occur during the refractory periods. In order for this to occur, they need to be sensed. The events just do not affect LRI timing because they occur during the refractory period

CASE 5 (✷✷✷)

What mode(s) of pacing could produce this rhythm? (Assume ventricular based pacing and no retrograde P waves!)

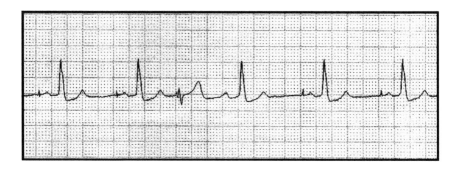

DDD or DDI

The LRI can be estimated between the atrial pacing spikes at the beginning or end of the strip. There is no atrial pacing spike at the end of the LRI after the PVC, which means that it must have been sensed and inhibited atrial pacing. Therefore AAI pacing is not possible and this must be a dual-chamber pacing mode.

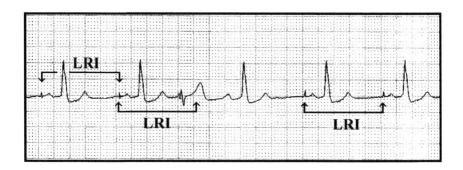

Next, the VA interval can be found by measuring backwards from an atrial pacing spike to an R wave. Measuring the VA interval forwards from the PVC (recall ventricular based pacing response to a PVC?!) shows that the subsequent P wave was sensed and inhibited atrial pacing at the end of the interval. Thus, because there is atrial pacing and sensing, DOO, VDD, and DVI pacing are not possible.

Is this DDD with a long AV interval, or DDI? This cannot be differentiated because it is not known whether the sensed P wave triggered an AV interval.

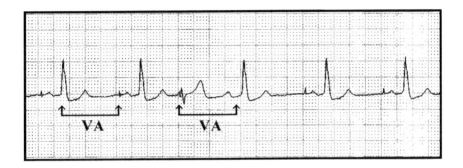

Case 6 (✸✸✸✸)

What mode(s) of pacing could produce this rhythm? (That's right, same rhythm but now assume pure atrial based pacing, a long AV interval and no retrograde P waves!)

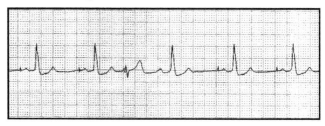

DDD, DDI, or DVI

The exact LRI can be measured between the atrial pacing spikes at the beginning or end of the strip. Again, there is no atrial pacing spike at the end of the LRI after the PVC, which means that it must have been sensed and inhibited atrial pacing. Therefore AAI pacing is not possible and this must be a dual-chamber pacing mode.

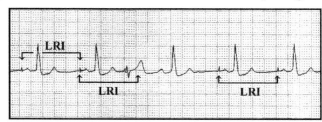

Next, there is no atrial pacing spike after measuring the LRI interval forward from the PVC (recall pure atrial based pacing response to a PVC?!). Therefore, either the P wave was sensed to inhibit atrial pacing as would happen with DDD or DDI, or it was not sensed and the sensed R wave inhibited atrial pacing as would happen with DVI. Again, because it is not known whether the P wave was sensed and triggered an AV interval, DDD versus DDI cannot be differentiated.

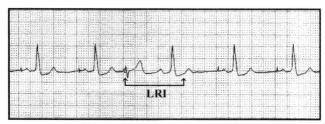

CASE 7 (✳✳)

A 48-year-old female is admitted to the coronary care unit (CCU) with an acute coronary syndrome. The medical team taking care of her wishes to know how her permanent pacemaker is programmed. Unfortunately, she does not know and does not carry a card with her programmed settings. The team presents you with this paced rhythm strip with PVC. What are the pacing mode, LRI and AV intervals?

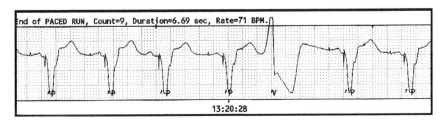

Bonus question!!!! What is the pacing base?

DDD 70 (857 ms)/200

PURE ATRIAL BASED

This is a dual-chamber pacing mode as evidenced by the atrial and ventricular pacing spikes. The AV interval and LRI can be measured at the beginning of the strip. VDD pacing is not possible because of the presence of atrial pacing. There is a sensed P wave with a triggered ventricular pacing spike at the end of the AV interval; therefore DDI, DVI, and DOO pacing are not possible. Thus, this must be DDD pacing!

The key to determining the pacing base comes from the sensed PVC. The pacemaker waits the *LRI* after it before pacing the atrium, which occurs with pure atrial based pacing.

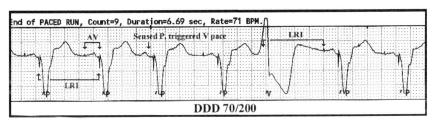

Chapter 19

Case Studies Part B

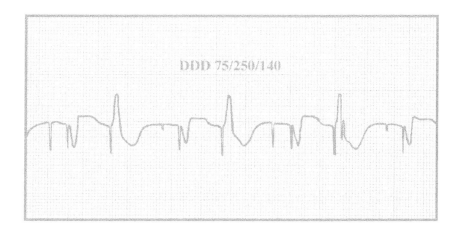

In this part the mode, LRI, and where applicable, AV interval and URI are given. The pacemaker function(s) may or may not be abnormal.

These cases are not necessarily meant to test one's knowledge, but are more so meant to further demonstrate the application of the basic timing intervals for troubleshooting potentially abnormal pacemaker rhythms. Each case also attempts to go beyond this by introducing common causes of the various pacing abnormalities.

The goal is to learn from each rhythm by applying the basic timing intervals, and at times refractory periods, and to determine the integrity of pacing system function.

CASE 8 (✱)

A 51-year-old male in the coronary care unit (CCU) had a temporary transvenous external VVI pacemaker inserted for significant sinus pauses while awaiting a permanent pacemaker system. The nurse taking care of the patient notices the following ECG rhythm strip and believes there to be a problem.

Is there a problem, and if so, what is it?

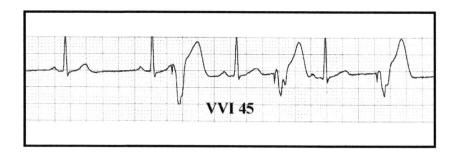

INTERMITTENT LOSS OF VENTRICULAR SENSING

There appears to be ventricular pacing occurring too close to native R waves on initial inspection. The first pacing spike even falls into the previous T wave! Measuring the lower rate interval (LRI) backwards from each pacing spike shows that only the first R wave is sensed.

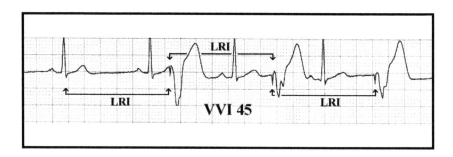

Chest radiography demonstrated that the pacing wire had moved in the ventricle.

Temporary transvenous pacemaker wires typically have no active mechanism for keeping them in place. Because of this it is not unusual for their position to change, a situation otherwise known as lead dislodgment. This can result in loss of sensing, pacing, or both. This is significant because loss of ventricular sensing with ventricular pacing into the T wave can very rarely cause ventricular fibrillation.

Management Solution: Reposition ventricular lead.

It is not unusual for the position of a temporary transvenous pacing wire to _____.

Ventricular pacing into the T wave can rarely cause _____ _____.

CHANGE
VENTRICULAR FIBRILLATION

Case 9 (✲)

A 68-year-old male with an AAI pacing system (LRI 80 beats per minute [bpm], atrial refractory period [ARP] 350 ms) had emergency coronary artery bypass graft surgery. On the first postoperative day, his surgeons wished to know whether the pacing system was still functioning correctly.

Is there a problem, and if so, what is it?

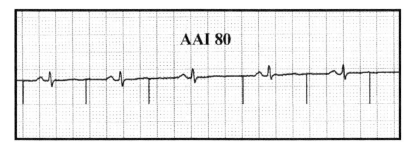

LOSS OF ATRIAL CAPTURE

The atrial pacing spikes occur outside of native refractory periods and do not capture. In order to determine if sensing is intact, the ARPs need to be superimposed after each pacing spike to see which P waves occur after them. Measuring the LRI backwards from the pacing spikes demonstrates that the only P wave outside of refractory is sensed.

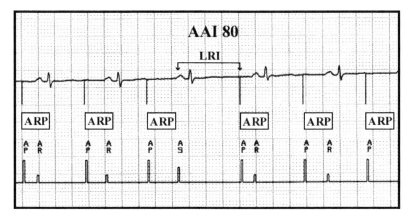

When a bypass surgery is performed a device called a "cannula" is inserted into the right atrial appendage. It is not unusual for a right atrial pacemaker lead to be damaged during the procedure or for there to be muscular inflammation at the cannula site. Inflammation can increase the pacing threshold.

In this case the atrial lead remained intact, so it is likely that atrial muscle inflammation caused the loss of capture. After time it may resolve and the threshold may improve.

Management Solution: Increase atrial pacing output. If capture absent or threshold remains too high, then revise atrial lead.

Bypass surgery can ＿＿＿＿＿ an atrial pacemaker lead or ＿＿＿＿＿ the atrial pacing threshold.

DAMAGE, INCREASE

CASE 10 (*)

A 50-year-old male with a VVI pacing system implanted for intermittent complete heart block (CHB) has the following rhythm strip during a trans-telephonic monitoring test.

Is there a problem, and if so, what is it?

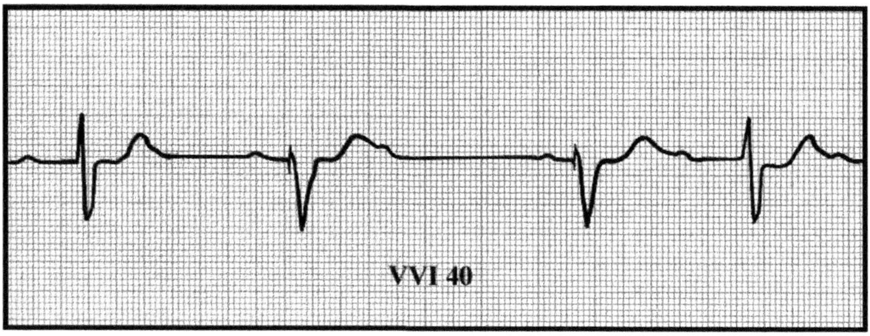

T WAVE OVERSENSING

The interval between the ventricular pacing spikes is greater than the LRI. When the LRI is measured backwards from the second pacing spike, the point of ventricular sensing that started this LRI falls into the previous T wave.

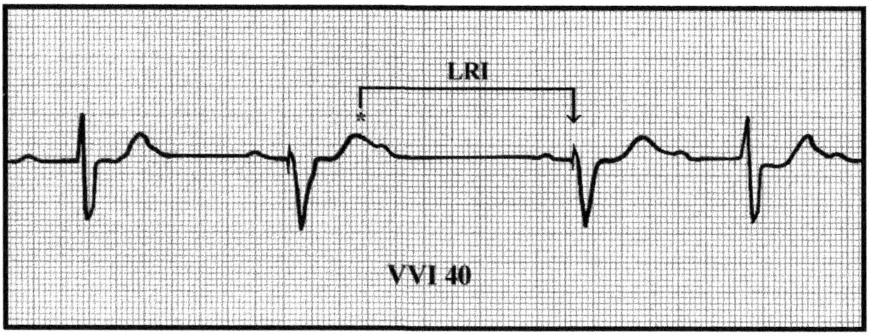

T wave oversensing can result in intervals longer than expected between events. Hysteresis can also produce an interval longer than the LRI, yet only after a sensed event.

Management Solution: Decrease ventricular sensitivity.

T wave oversensing can result in an interval between events that is _____ than expected.

LONGER

Case 11 (✻)

A 33-year-old female with a VVI pacing system is started on flecainide for a history of paroxysmal atrial fibrillation (AF). One month later a trans-telephonic pacemaker test is done. The ventricular refractory period (VRP) is 350 ms.

Is there a problem, and if so, what is it?

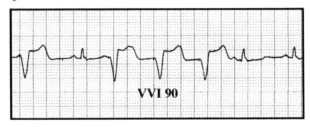

INTERMITTENT LOSS OF VENTRICULAR CAPTURE

On the strip there are two intervals between events that are greater than the LRI. Measuring the LRI between them identifies the ventricular pacing spikes that do not capture.

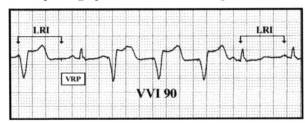

Chest radiography subsequently demonstrated no change in the appropriate ventricular lead position, and no evidence of lead fracture. Lead impedance was also measured and found to be unchanged and within normal limits.

The medication flecainide can increase pacing threshold. Amiodarone and propafenone are other medicines that can do this as well. Threshold can even increase to the point where discontinuation of the medication may be necessary to prevent premature battery depletion.

Management Solution: Increase pacemaker output. Follow pacing threshold closely.

Medications that can increase pacing threshold are _____, _____, and _____.

FLECAINIDE, AMIODARONE, PROPAFENONE

CASE 12 (✱)

A 30-year-old male with a unipolar VVI pacing system implanted for congenital CHB presents to the emergency room (ER) after falling through the ice of a frozen lake.

The ER physician wishes to know whether the pacemaker is working properly. What is happening?

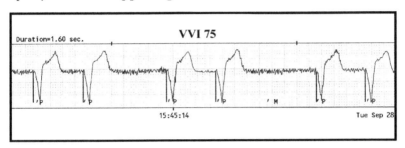

MYOPTENTIAL OVERSENSING

There are intervals between the unipolar ventricular pacing spikes that are greater than the LRI. There is also significant baseline "noise" most likely from the patient shivering. When the LRI is measured backwards from the delayed ventricular pacing spikes it is seen that the points of ventricular sensing that started these LRIs occurs within the "noise." The "noise" is the skeletal muscle potentials (myopotentials) intermittently sensed by the unipolar pacing system.

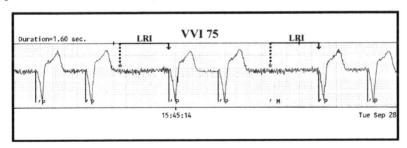

Electrical activity of a large enough size and occurring anywhere between the pacemaker generator and the pacemaker lead tip has the potential for being sensed and inhibiting pacing by a unipolar pacing system.

In addition to myopotentials, the signal from an electric cautery knife ("bovi") can also inappropriately inhibit pacing. Such sensing is much rarer with a bipolar pacing configuration simply because the area within which it looks to sense (between the electrodes within the heart) is much smaller than that of a unipolar pacing system.

Some pacemakers will allow programming to either a unipolar or bipolar sensing and/or pacing configuration so long as a bipolar lead has been implanted.

Management Solution: Decrease ventricular sensitivity. If available, reprogram sensing configuration to bipolar.

Myopotentials can be of sufficient size to be _____, especially by a _____ pacing system.

SENSED, UNIPOLAR

CASE 13 (❋)

An 80-year-old demented female is admitted to the intensive care until (ICU) with severe pulmonary fibrosis and respiratory distress. She also has a VVI pacing system implanted. Her family wishes no aggressive measures to be taken in her care. A few hours after admission she stops breathing and her ECG rhythm changes dramatically over the course of a few minutes.

What happened?

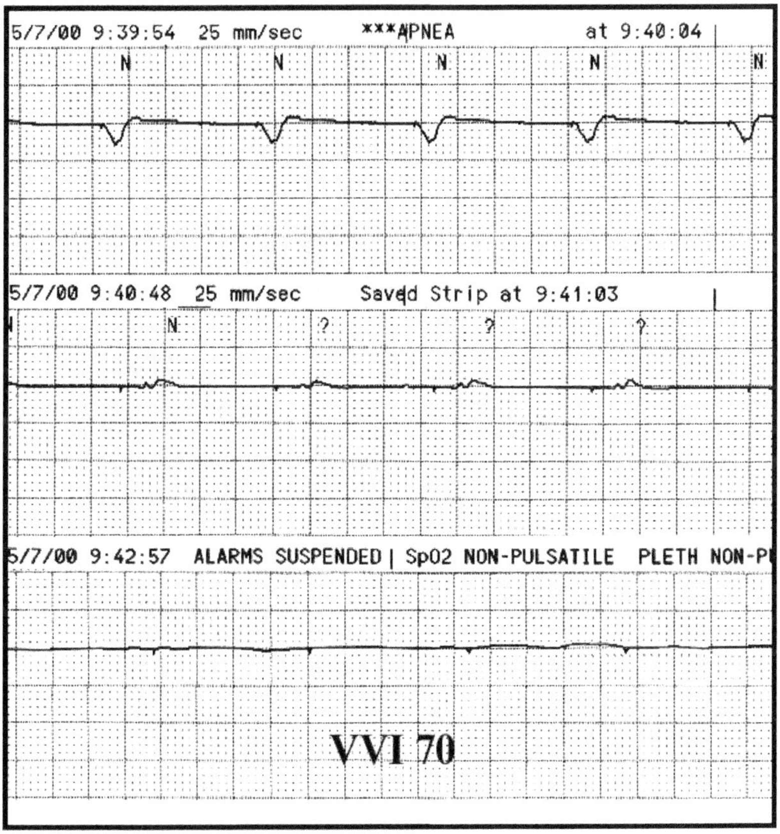

LOSS OF VENTRICULAR CAPTURE

Because she stopped breathing a severe acidosis developed. This caused her heart to eventually become unexcitable by the pacemaker spikes.

The second strip demonstrates the initial changes in the heart's excitability as the time between each pacemaker spike and the actual R wave increased. This is a phenomenon called "latency." The R wave morphologies on this strip are also different because the acidosis changed the electrical characteristics of the heart tissue.

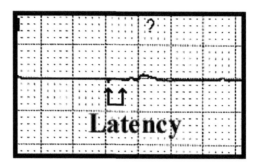

In addition to acidosis other nonpacemaker problems can affect the excitability of cardiac tissue. They include an elevated blood potassium, glucose or carbon dioxide level, a low oxygen level, and a myocardial infarction or fibrosis at the pacemaker lead attachment site.

Management Solution: Emergently reverse the cause of acidosis if possible.

The time between a pacemaker spike and the captured cardiac signal is called _____.

Factors that may affect cardiac excitability include _____, the levels of _____, _____, _____ _____, _____, and _____ _____ or _____ at the pacemaker lead attachment site.

LATENCY
ACIDOSIS, POTASSIUM, GLUCOSE, CARBON DIOXIDE, OXYGEN, MYOCARDIAL INFARCTION, FIBROSIS

CASE 14 (✴)

A 32-year-old male presents to the emergency room complaining of intermittent "weakness, lightheadedness, shortness of breath, and fullness in his neck" for the past 2 weeks. He has a history of a permanent pacemaker placed in another state for a "slow heartbeat" as well as two episodes of AF at 19 and 26 years of age. At the time you initially see him he is asymptomatic.

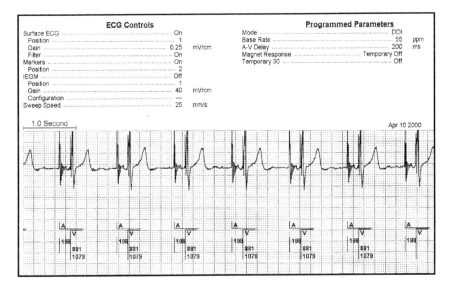

During evaluation he begins complaining of his symptoms and a new rhythm is noted. The postventricular atrial refractory period (PVARP) is 250 ms.

Is there a pacemaker problem?

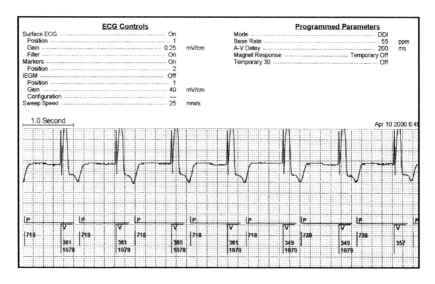

NORMAL DDI FUNCTION

There is no problem. The ventricular pacing spikes initially occurring simultaneously with normally conducted R waves begin capturing and cause retrograde atrial conduction. Each retrograde P wave occurs outside of the PVARP, is sensed, and inhibits atrial pacing. Atrial sensing then *does not* initiate an atrioventricular (AV) interval, as expected in the DDI mode, and ventricular pacing at the lower rate results.

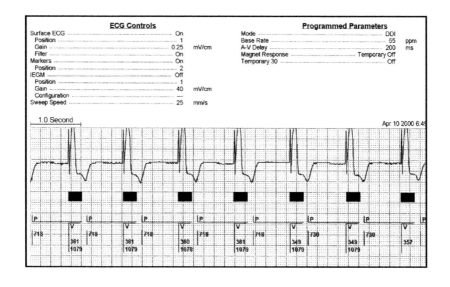

Symptoms such as those described by this patient have been attributed to ventricular pacing and included in the "*pacemaker syndrome.*" It is a constellation of symptoms thought to be caused by the hemodynamic changes resulting from the loss of AV synchrony. The symptoms can be profound enough to cause significant disability, and may result in the need to upgrade a ventricular pacemaker to a dual-chamber pacing system that will maintain AV synchrony.

Management Solutions: A) Program pacing mode to DDD with mode switching (given history of AF), if available, and increase PVARP to prevent pacemaker-mediated tachycardia (PMT). B) Consider DDD mode if no mode switching available given rarity of AF, and increase PVARP to prevent PMT.

Ventricular pacing can result in symptoms that are termed the ——————— ———————.

PACEMAKER SYNDROME

CASE 15 (✻✻✻✻)

A 67-year-old female had a DDD pacing system implanted for CHB. On the morning after implantation her ECG rhythm strip was felt to be abnormal.

Is there a problem, and if so, what is it?

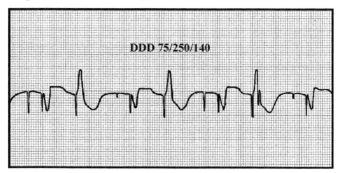

ATRIAL LEAD DISLODGMENT TO THE VENTRICLE

In this example there do not appear to be any P waves after what appear to be atrial pacing spikes. This is the first clue that something is not quite right. There are also two different captured R wave morphologies, which is the second clue. The pacing spikes with each of the first captured R wave morphologies occur at the end of the AV interval, thus identifying these spikes as ventricular. The pacing spikes with each of the second captured R wave morphologies do not appear to occur after any identifiable P wave when the AV interval is measured backwards from them. They do occur at exactly the end of the ventriculoatrial (VA) interval when measured from the previous ventricular pacing spikes. This identifies the pacing spike with each of the second R wave morphologies as atrial. Chest radiography showed both pacing leads to be in the ventricle.

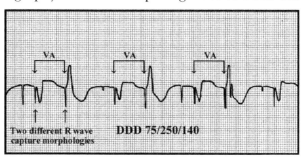

Atrial lead dislodgment is one of the most frequently encountered early postimplant pacing system problems. When this occurs atrial pacing and/or sensing function may be intermittent or completely absent. On occasion the atrial lead tip will cross into the ventricle and pace the ventricle!

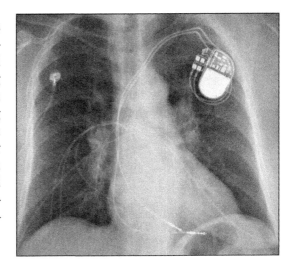

Management Solution: Reposition the atrial lead.

One of the most frequently seen pacing system problems in the immediate postimplant period is ————— ————— —————.

Measuring ————— the AV or VA interval from paced events helps to identify the event that initiated the interval.

ATRIAL LEAD DISLODGMENT
BACKWARDS

CASE 16 (✶✶✶✶✶✶)

A 54-year-old male with paroxysmal AF was having a DDI pacing system implanted for symptomatic bradycardia. As the implanting surgeon was closing the patient's pacemaker pocket, the pacemaker engineer assisting the procedure noticed the pacemaker rhythm seen below, and suggested to the surgeon that he stop to investigate the pacing system for a "problem." After some further debate the surgeon did so.

Is there a problem, and if so, what is it and what might the engineer have suggested the surgeon do?

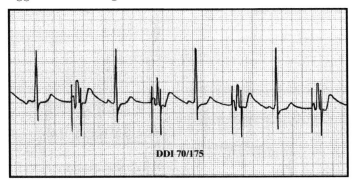

PACEMAKER LEADS CONNECTED TO THE WRONG PORTS IN THE PACEMAKER

The engineer noticed that the atrial pacing spikes were capturing the ventricle! His first suggestion was to fluoroscopically look at the pacing system to rule out an atrial lead dislodged to the ventricle, or coronary sinus (this is a large vein that drains into the right atrium but is near enough to the ventricle that the ventricle could possibly be captured). After the leads were confirmed to be in

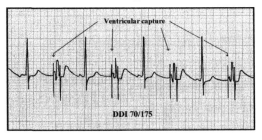

their appropriate posi-tions in the heart the engineer suggested that the atrial lead was plugged into the ventricular lead port in the pacemaker, and ventricular lead was plugged into the atrial lead port in the pacemaker. The surgeon reluctantly opened the pacemaker pocket and found this to be so. (Another way of confirming this would have been to program the pacemaker VVI and note atrial capture and sensing.)

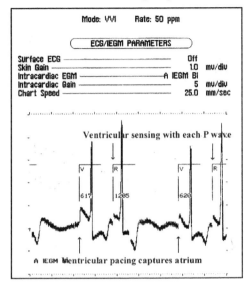

Near the plug of each pacemaker lead, a serial number is printed. It is helpful to note the serial number of each pacing lead as they are being implanted, so that the identity of each lead can be confirmed when plugging them into the pacemaker. This problem rarely happens, but is easily avoided by performing this exercise.

Management Solution: Plug the pacemaker leads into the proper position in the pacemaker.

An atrial lead dislodged to the ventricle or the coronary sinus and an _____ lead plugged into the _____ lead port in the pacemaker are causes of ventricle capture by an atrial pacing spike.

ATRIAL, VENTRICULAR

CASE 17 (✳✳✳)

An 81-year-old male with a DDD pacing system implanted for sinus bradycardia has the following rhythm strip recorded while undergoing a trans-telephonic pacemaker evaluation.

Is there a problem, and if so, what is it?

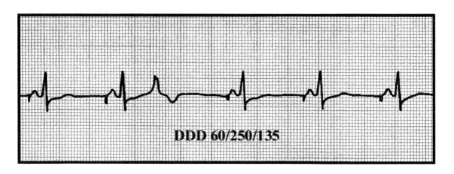

DDD 60/250/135

NORMAL FUNCTION WITH A "PURE" ATRIAL BASED PACING SYSTEM
T WAVE OVERSENSING WITH A "MODIFIED" ATRIAL BASED PACING SYSTEM

It needs to be determined what the pacing base is for a proper diagnosis. It is atrial because the atrial pacing interval is maintained at the lower rate. Recall that with a "pure" atrial based pacing system a premature ventricular contraction (PVC) inhibits both atrial and ventricular pacing, and waits the *LRI* before pacing the atrium. In this example the atrial pacing spike occurs at exactly the LRI after the PVC. Thus this would be normal function.

With a "modified" atrial based pacing system a PVC inhibits both atrial and ventricular pacing for that cycle, and waits the *VA* interval before pacing the atrium. The interval between the PVC and the subsequent atrial pacing spike is longer than this. Measuring the VA interval backwards from the atrial pacing spike that follows the PVC places the point of ventricular sensing that initiated this VA interval in the T wave of the PVC. This is not normal function.

The T wave can on occasion have a large enough signal such that it is sensed by the ventricular lead, as long as it occurs after the VRP.

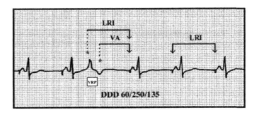

Management Solutions: A) No change is indicated for normal pure atrial based pacing. B) Decrease the ventricular sensitivity, or increase the VRP for modified atrial based pacing.

The interval that is initiated when a PVC is sensed with modified atrial based pacing is the _____ interval, and with pure atrial based pacing is the _____.

The interval that is initiated when a PVC is sensed with ventricular based pacing is the _____ interval.

T wave oversensing can result in an interval before the next pacing spike that is _____ than expected.

VA, LRI
VA
LONGER

CASE 18 (✷✷✷)

Three weeks after having a DDD pacing system implanted for sick sinus syndrome a 25-year-old male was asked to return to the pacemaker clinic because of an abnormal pacemaker telephone test. After questioning the patient it was noted that he had been rowing a boat a few days prior to the telephone test.

The pacing base is ventricular, and the VRP and PVARP are 260 ms and 325 ms, respectively. What pacemaker function(s) are absent/present on this rhythm strip, and what is the likely cause of any abnormality?

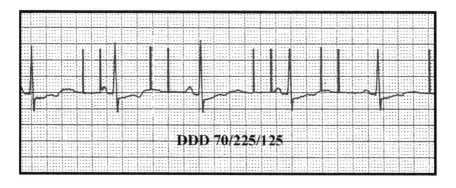

DDD 70/225/125

ATRIAL CAPTURE → ABSENT
VENTRICULAR CAPTURE → ABSENT
ATRIAL SENSING → UNKNOWN
VENTRICULAR SENSING → PRESENT
ATRIAL AND VENTRICULAR LEAD DISLODGMENT

The most obvious abnormality is that there is no capture by either of the pacing leads. Next, before a determination of proper sensing can be made one needs to superimpose the VRPs and PVARPs onto the strip after the ventricular pacing spikes. Measuring the VA interval backwards from each atrial pacing spike shows that each R wave outside of refractory is sensed.

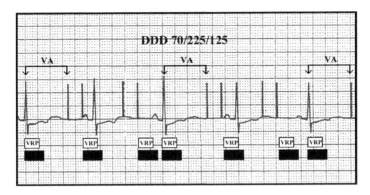

Only the last P wave on the strip falls outside of the PVARP. If both this P and the following R wave are sensed, atrial and ventricular pacing are inhibited. The VA interval follows the R wave and ends with an atrial pacing spike. On the other hand if the P wave is not sensed, the following R wave is sensed, with both atrial and ventricular pacing being inhibited (the R wave is sensed as a PVC). Again the VA interval is initiated and ends with an atrial pacing spike. Thus, the ECG strip looks the same whether the P wave is sensed or not.

What was the likely cause of this? Given that the patient performed an activity that resulted in excessive tugging on the leads before they were properly healed (usually takes about 6 weeks), suspicion for lead dislodgment was very high. Chest radiography confirmed the diagnosis.

Management Solution: Reposition both leads.

It takes approximately _____ after implantation before pacing leads are properly healed.

6 WEEKS

CASE 19 (✳✳✳✳)

An 80-year-old female with a DDD pacing system implanted for sick sinus syndrome presents to the emergency room because of palpitations. You are asked to evaluate the patient for a "pacemaker malfunction."

Is there a problem, and if so, what is it?

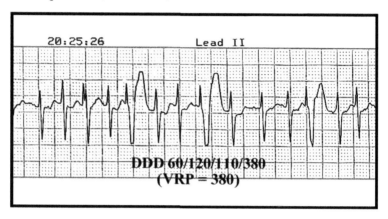

TRACKING OF AF

On first look it appears that there are ventricular pacing spikes occurring too close to the previous R waves and that the underlying rhythm is rapid AF. The key to understanding this rhythm is to measure the upper rate interval (URI) backwards from the ventricular pacing spikes to see what events initiated them. When all of the VRPs are plotted, it is seen that many of the R waves fall into the VRP, and that none of the ventricular pacing spikes occurs too early.

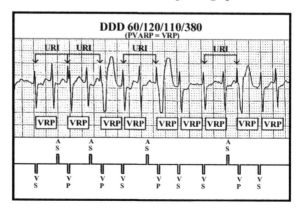

When a drug is administered to keep the AF from making the native ventricular rate so fast, ventricular pacing still occurs at the upper rate limit (URL). This is because atrial sensing during AF frequently occurs just after the end of each PVARP.

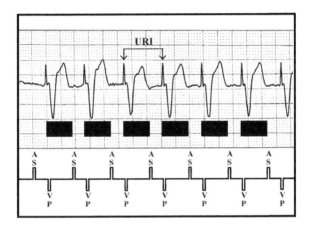

Management Solution: Program mode switching on if available, or program mode to VVI.

Upper rate ventricular pacing in the DDD pacing mode without visible P waves is often due to _____.

AF

CASE 20 (✱)

Three months after having a DDD pacing system implanted for sick sinus syndrome a 77-year-old female presents to clinic for her first postimplant office visit. A rhythm strip is initially obtained and a pacing problem is suspected.

The atrial and ventricular pacing outputs are 0.5 ms and 5 V, and the atrial and ventricular sensitivities are 0.5 mV and 2.5 mV, respectively. Multiple measurements of lead impedance are stable and unchanged from implant.

Is the suspicion correct, and if so, what is the problem?

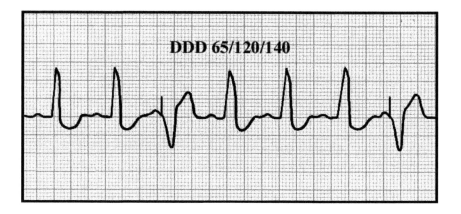

INTERMITTENT LOSS OF ATRIAL SENSING

Only the third and the last P waves are followed by ventricular pacing spikes at the end of the AV interval. The others are followed by native R waves at an interval greater than the AV interval. Either there is intermittent loss of ventricular pacing or the P waves are not sensed and the subsequent R waves occur before the VA interval (803 ms) ends and inhibit both atrial and ventricular pacing. Intermittent loss of ventricular pacing output is unlikely given the normal, and unchanged lead impedance measurements.

Pacing thresholds are found to be only slightly elevated from those at implant, however the P wave amplitude varies between 0.3 mV and 1 mV (P wave amplitude at implant was 1.5 mV). Lead impedances are essentially unchanged from implant. Marker channels demonstrate the intermittent loss of atrial sensing. Chest radiography also shows appropriate lead positions unchanged from implant.

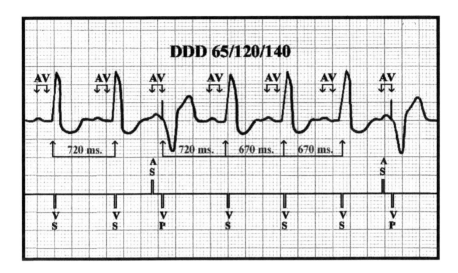

It is not unusual for pacing and sensing thresholds to rise in the postimplant period (about 6 weeks). This occurs because of a fibrotic healing process at the lead tip-cardiac interface.

Management Solution: Increase atrial sensitivity. If undersensing not resolved with adequate safety margin, then reposition atrial lead.

Pacing and sensing threshold may _____ over the post-implant period.

INCREASE

Case 21 (✱✱✱)

Shortly after receiving a DDD pacing system for sick sinus syndrome, an 80-year-old female has the following rhythm strip on telemetry.

Is there a problem, and if so, what is it?

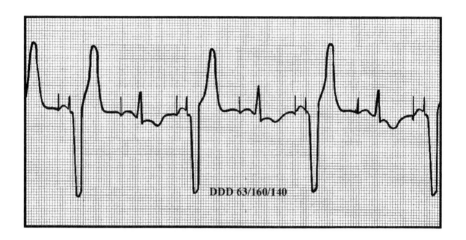

DDD 63/160/140

CROSSTALK

Two things are immediately evident on first inspection. There are no ventricular pacing spikes despite an absence of ventricular activity during the AV interval every other cycle. Second, the A-A interval is shortened every other cycle. When the VA interval is measured backwards from the shortened atrial pacing spikes it is noted that ventricular sensing occurs just after the previous atrial pacing spike. This is crosstalk!

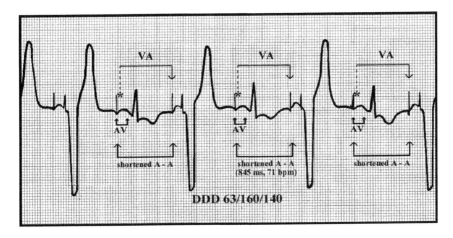

DDD 63/160/140

Management Solution: Decrease atrial output and/or ventricular sensitivity, and/or increase ventricular blanking period.

Crosstalk frequently occurs with a _____ atrial pacing output, and can cause a shortened _____ pacing interval.

HIGH, A–A

CASE 22 (✲)

A 42-year-old female aerobics instructor with a DDD pacing system implanted 8 years ago presents to the pacemaker clinic for complaints of fatigue and weakness that began during class 2 days ago. The following rhythm strip is obtained. Safety pacing is programmed on, and the VRP is 400 ms.

What is the problem?

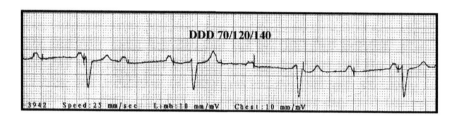

LOSS OF VENTRICULAR CAPTURE AND POSSIBLE LOSS OF SENSING

There are ventricular pacing spikes without capture at the end of the AV interval with each P wave. The underlying rhythm is CHB, which would explain the complaints of weakness and fatigue.

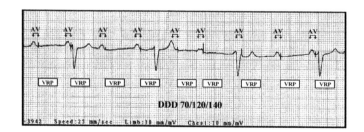

Only the third R wave falls outside of the VRP. Because safety pacing is programmed "on" this R wave should elicit an early safety pacing spike if it is sensed. It is hard to tell given the short AV interval that is programmed, but it may be likely that it is not sensed.

What caused the loss of capture? The ventricular lead's measured impedance was greater than 4000 Ω. This information, coupled with the clinical history raised the suspicion of a ventricular lead fracture that was subsequently confirmed with chest radiography. Suspicion of lead dislodgment was also considered, yet would have been highly unusual given that the lead had been in place for 8 years.

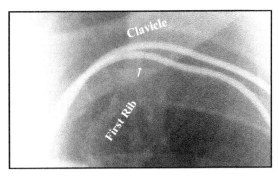

Most lead fractures occur at the junction of the first rib and the clavicle where these bones tend to crush the lead(s) between them as it enters the venous system. It usually takes years of this lead injury to result in a fracture. Lead fractures can also commonly occur at the site where the lead has been sutured in the pocket. *Management Solution:* Replace the ventricular lead.

Lead fractures most commonly occur at the _____ _____ _____ junction.

FIRST RIB, CLAVICULAR

CASE 23 (✱)

A 43-year-old male with sick sinus syndrome has a DDD pacing system implanted. The morning after his procedure the medical team rounding on the patient notes him to be complaining of intermittent sharp pain and twitching in the left lower chest and brings the following magnet rhythm strip to your attention. He is otherwise stable. After examining the patient and analyzing the system with the pacemaker programmer you agree that there is a problem.

What is the problem and the likely cause?

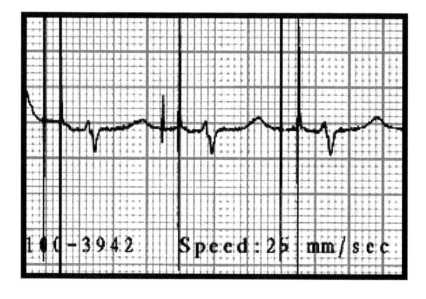

LOSS OF VENTRICULAR CAPTURE
VENTRICULAR LEAD PERFORATION

The loss of ventricular capture is fairly obvious. What is more concerning in this case are the accompanying complaints of chest

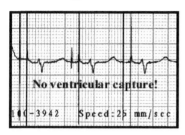

pain and intercostal muscle twitching (pacing capture of chest muscle!). All of this information combined together should produce a high suspicion for lead perforation. Chest radiography demonstrated advancement of the ventricular lead beyond the cardiac silhouette.

Perforation of a ventricular pacing lead can result in the lead tip either advancing to the left ventricle, or directly out the right ventricle to the pericardial space and beyond. Lead tips in the left ventricle may also result in loss of ventricular capture, or capture with a right bundle branch block (RBBB) morphology. Perforation to the pericardial space can also cause cardiac tamponade. This is an emergent

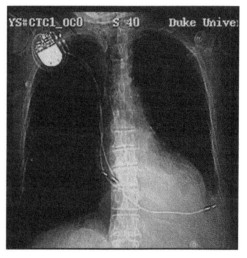

medical condition that causes blood to escape into the pericardial space outside the heart and may be deadly if not promptly treated.

Management Solution: Pull back ventricular lead with careful attention to hemodynamic status.

A pacemaker lead can perforate to the _____ _____ or _____ _____.

LEFT VENTRICLE, PERICARDIAL SPACE

CASE 24 (✳✳)

While evaluating a pacemaker patient for palpitations the following rhythm strip is noted. The PVARP is 200 ms.

What is the rhythm, and how can it be fixed?

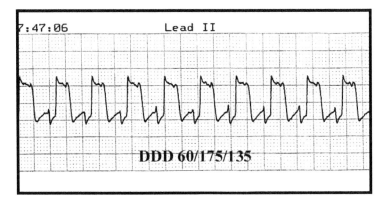

PMT

The ventricle is paced at upper rate. There are also P waves that occur after the PVARP and are buried in each of the paced ventricular complexes. When a magnet is placed over the pacemaker the rhythm breaks clinching the diagnosis of PMT.

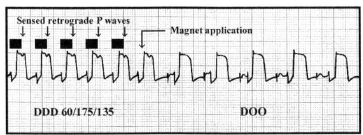

PMT should be suspected when the ventricle is persistently paced at the URL and when there are identifiable P waves before each paced ventricular complex. If there were no visible P waves, tracking of AF might be likely.

Management Solution: Increase the PVARP.

Persistent pacing at the URL could be due to either _____ or _____.

PMT, AF

CASE 25 (✻✻✻)

You receive a call from the telemetry floor that your pacemaker patient is having frequent "pauses" on the monitor. The PVARP is 325 ms.

Is there a problem, and if so, what is it?

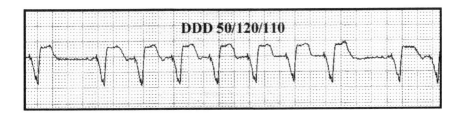

NORMAL UPPER RATE WENCKEBACH BEHAVIOR

Besides the "pauses," the other remarkable feature is that the pacemaker is at upper rate probably from tracking sinus tachycardia. P waves are evident and the AV intervals following them progressively increase until a P wave falls into the PVARP and is not sensed. The "pause" then occurs until the next P wave is sensed, repeating the sequence.

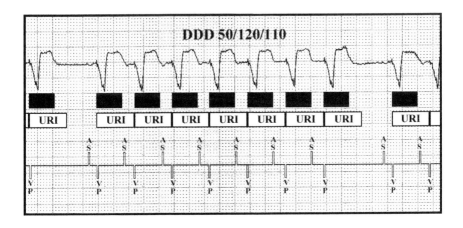

Why is this not intermittent PMT? With PMT the interval between the retrograde P wave and the subsequent ventricular pacing spike typically remains fixed, which does not happen here (gets progressively longer). Also it is clear from the "pauses" that the P waves are not generated by retrograde conduction with ventricular pacing.

Some pacemakers have a function that can prevent such pauses from happening during high pacing rates. They prevent this by pacing the atrium when it is determined that a significant interval has passed after a ventricular pacing output without sensing a P wave (i.e., as would happen when a P wave falls into the PVARP during upper rate Wenckebach behavior). This type of function is sometimes referred to as "rate smoothing."

Management Solution: Treat the tachycardia, and/or its cause. Decrease the PVARP or program on a "rate smoothing" type function, if available, if this happens and causes symptoms during exertion.

Upper rate Wenckebach behavior can cause _____ in P wave tracking.

"PAUSES"

CASE 26 (✳✳✳)

While evaluating a pacemaker patient in the electrophysiology laboratory you place a magnet over the device and the following occurs.

What happened?

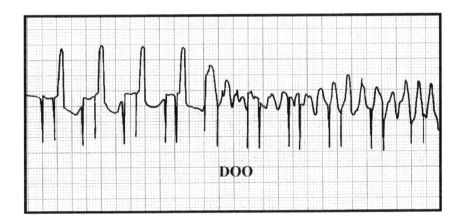

DOO

VENTRICULAR FIBRILLATION

There is a PVC within which a ventricular pacing spike occurs. The pacing spike may have happened at a critical time in the PVC and induced ventricular fibrillation (VF) as opposed to the PVC occurring at a critical time in the T wave prior to it and inducing VF.

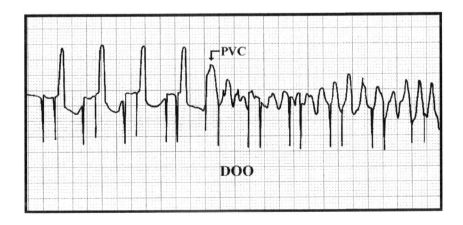

PVC

DOO

VF induced by an asynchronous ventricular pacing spike is almost unheard of. Personal experience includes this example as one of three possible in 12 years time.

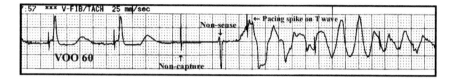

Management Solution: Immediate defibrillation. There is no prevention that can be taken with magnet placement. Otherwise the permanent pacing mode should include ventricular sensing!

VF caused by asynchronous ventricular pacing into a critical portion of a native QRS complex is extremely _____.

RARE

CASE 27 (✷✷✷)

A 73-year-old female with a dual-chamber implanted cardi-overter-defibrillator (ICD) and history of kidney failure presents to the emergency room with weakness. The following rhythm strip is recorded.

What is the problem?

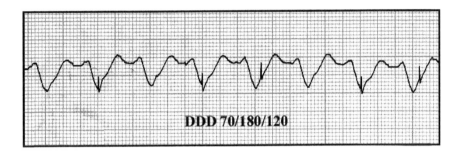

INTERMITTENT LOSS OF VENTRICULAR SENSING FROM SEVERE HYPERKALEMIA

Pacing spikes appear in the middle of several QRS complexes so ventricular sensing is intermittent. The third and fifth pacing spikes are ventricular (the other pacing spikes may also be) as they occur above the lower rate. The P waves that are tracked are not clearly seen.

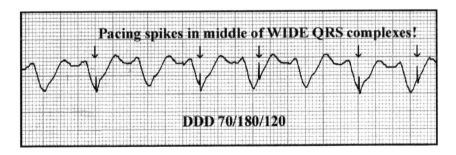

The patient had an acute worsening of renal failure and had a potassium level of 8 mEq/dL (*really* high). This caused an alteration of the ventricular electrogram (EGM) such that the R waves were only intermittently sensed. Treatment of the elevated potassium without any pacemaker adjustments resulted in normalization of the underlying rhythm and pacing function (P waves still not easily seen!).

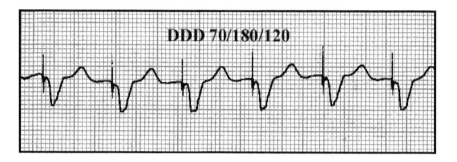

Management Solution: Treat elevated potassium level.

An elevated potassium level can alter the _____.

EGM

CASE 28 (✻)

A 71-year-old male with hypersensitive carotid sinus syndrome displays the following rhythm strip while being evaluated in your office.

Is there a problem, and if so, what is it?

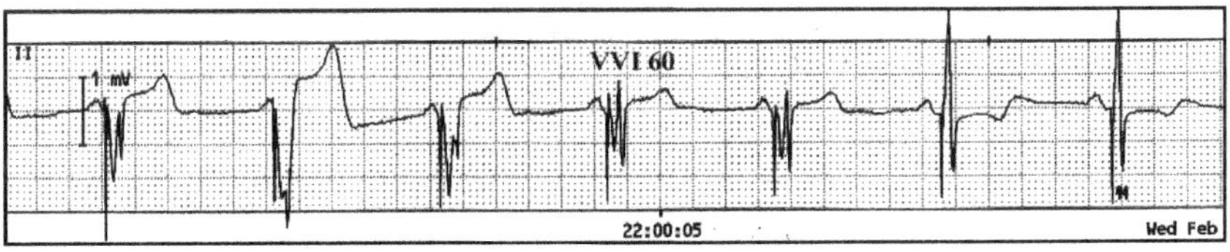

NORMAL VVI FUNCTION

Beats 1 and 3 through 5 display ventricular fusion. The second beat is a capture beat and the last two beats are native.

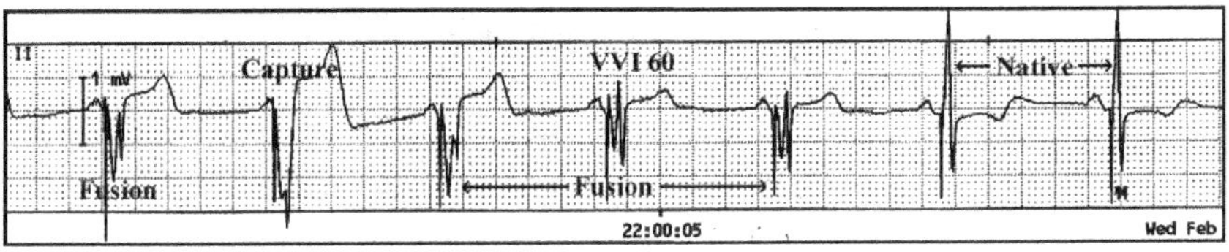

Ventricular pacing spikes appear at the onset of the two native beats. This is not from a loss of ventricular sensing. The cardiac tissue underlying the ventricular lead did not have enough time to generate an EGM of sufficient size to be sensed and inhibit pacing by the time the LRI timed out. The tissue at that instance is also refractory from capture due to native conduction.

Management Solution: None needed.

Ventricular fusion is a ________ occurrence.

NORMAL

CASE 29 (✳✳✳✳)

A 53-year-old male has just completed coronary bypass surgery and has a temporary external pacemaker (an older model). The nurse taking care of the patient brings you this rhythm strip and is concerned about a malfunction.

What's going on?

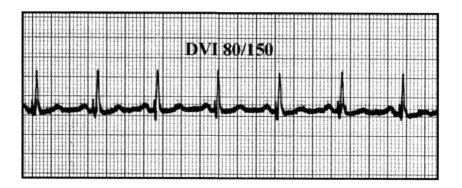

NORMAL DVI FUNCTION WITH VENTRICULAR BASED PACING

Each pacing spike occurs at exactly the VA interval and thus is atrial. (Remember, there is no atrial sensing in the DVI mode.) Measuring the VA interval (LRI–AVI; 750 ms–150 ms) backwards from the pacing spikes reveals the point of ventricular sensing that started the VA interval. Because the atrial pacing spikes occur at an interval shorter (670 ms) than the LRI (750 ms), the pacing base must be ventricular. Atrial based pacing would have maintained the A-A pacing interval at 750 ms. Why weren't there any safety pacing spikes with each R wave sensed so early in the AV interval? Older models of temporary external pacemakers do not have safety pacing!

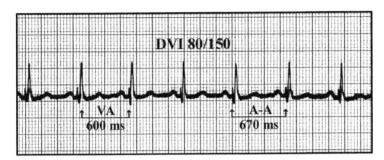

Management Solution: None needed. If atrial sensing desired then change mode to DDD.

With the DVI pacing mode there is no atrial _____.

With ventricular based pacing the atrium _____ be paced faster than the programmed lower rate.

SENSING
CAN

Case 30 (✱✱✱)

A 20-year-old male has an implantable defibrillator for a history of sudden cardiac death. When playing tennis he receives a shock from the device without any warning. While he is in the emergency room for evaluation, you interrogate the device and are able to analyze the ventricular EGM surrounding the event.

What happened?

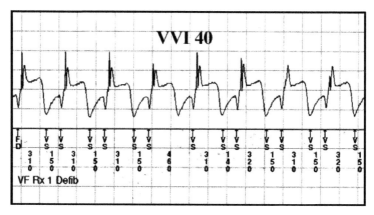

T WAVE OVERSENSING

The marker channel shows frequent T wave oversensing on the ventricular EGM.

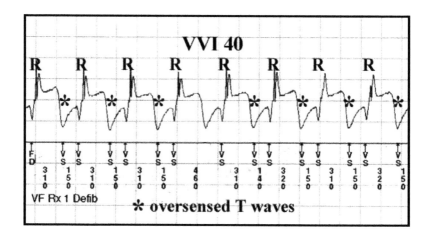

An implantable defibrillator may deliver therapy (i.e., overdrive pacing or an internal shock) based on sensing a rapid ventricular rhythm in addition to treating bradyarrhythmias with pacing. It may rarely happen that the T wave may be of such sufficient amplitude on a ventricular EGM that it is interpreted by the implanted device as an R wave. In the instance above this resulted in the patient being inappropriately shocked for what was sinus tachycardia.

Management Solution: Decrease ventricular sensitivity.*

_____ waves may be oversensed on a _____ EGM if they are of sufficient amplitude.

T, VENTRICULAR

---

*Consult the electrophysiology attending first. Decreasing ventricular sensitivity too much may cause even the R waves to not be sensed, which would be bad during a real ventricular tachyarrhythmia (i.e., the device might not recognize the rhythm and treat it!). Rarely the ventricular defibrillator lead might even need to be repositioned to minimize T waves on the EGM.

CASE 31 (✳✳✳✳)

A 71-year-old male with a dual-chamber pacemaker implanted 1 day ago for CHB has the following rhythm strip. Multiple readings of ventricular lead impedance show it to be greater than 2500 Ω.

What is the problem?

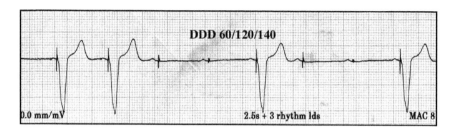

INTERMITTENT LOSS OF VENTRICULAR CAPTURE DUE TO A LOOSE SET SCREW

The ventricular pacing spikes without capture following sensed P waves are fairly obvious. There is also variable size to the pacing spikes.

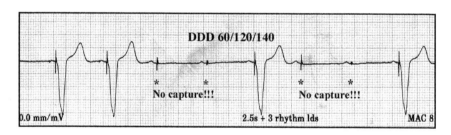

Loss of ventricular capture so soon after implant should raise the suspicion of an inappropriately programmed ventricular pacing output (i.e., right at pacing threshold or lower), an elevated pacing threshold, a dislodged ventricular lead, and a loose set screw. Variable size of the pacing spikes is consistent with an incomplete break in the pacemaker circuit, and is more suggestive of a dislodged lead or loose set screw. A fractured pacemaker lead, which could also result in loss of capture, an elevated lead impedance, and variable pacing spike size, is unheard of in my experience on the first day post implant.

Evaluation included a chest X-ray with no change in lead positioning from that at implant and an appropriately programmed pacing output. Given the intermittent ventricular pacing capture with low pacing outputs, variable pacemaker spike size, and persistent elevation in lead impedance readings a loose set screw was most likely. Opening the pacemaker pocket in the electrophysiology lab demonstrated the loose set screw.

Management Solution: Tighten the set screw.

Intermittent or no pacing capture with a greatly _____ lead impedance early after implant should raise the suspicion of a _____ set screw.

ELEVATED, LOOSE

CASE 32 (✸✸✸)

A 91-year-old female with a dual-chamber pacemaker implanted 10 years ago for sick sinus syndrome presents with complaint of an irregular heartbeat. The following rhythm strip is obtained.

What is happening?

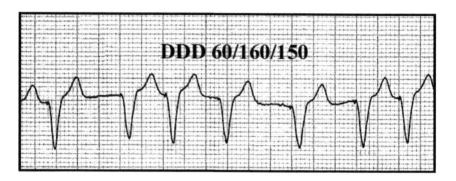

INTERMITTENT UNDERSENSING OF AF

The pacemaker is tracking at irregularly irregular intervals, with a few at upper rate. Also there are no identifiable P waves. This is virtually diagnostic of an underlying rhythm of AF.

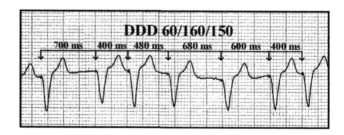

Persistent ventricular pacing at the URL with no identifiable P waves should raise the suspicion of an underlying rhythm of AF. This is because atrial fibrillatory waves are often sensed right after the PVARP. It may happen though that even with maximal atrial sensitivity the fibrillatory waves are so small as to only be intermittently sensed. This may lead to an irregularly irregular ventricular paced rhythm.

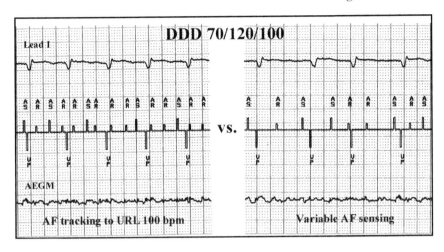

Wouldn't mode switching have been effective in this case? Automatic mode switching would not as it relies upon consistent sensing of atrial fibrillatory waves in order to make the switch to a nontracking mode.

Management Solution: If mode switching is not available or not effective with increased atrial sensitivity then reprogram mode to VVI(R) until possible cardioversion.

An irregularly irregular ventricular paced rhythm with no identifiable P waves is virtually diagnostic of _____.

AF

CASE 33 (✳✳)

You are called to the emergency room for a "pacemaker malfunction" in a 40-year-old male with congenital CHB. The emergency room physician had astutely checked the patient's records prior to calling you finding that the lower rate had been programmed to 60 pulses per minute (ppm) not 1 week ago in clinic, and noted now that the heart rate was 51 bpm with no pacing seen! You evaluate the pacemaker and find this to be appropriate for how it is programmed, and find no T wave oversensing.

How is this possible?

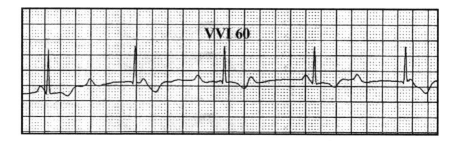

NORMAL FUNCTION WITH HYSTERESIS

The pacemaker also had hysteresis programmed to 50 bpm, which was not apparent in the record!

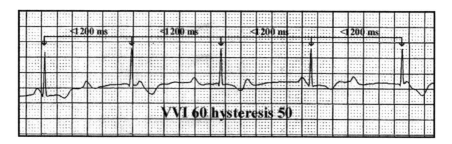

Hysteresis causes a pacemaker to wait a little longer than the LRI following a sensed event before it will pace. In this case it waited up to 1200 ms (50 ppm/60,000). Because each beat occurred at an interval slightly less than 1200 ms, no pacing was seen.

Management Solution: Document the presence of hysteresis in patient record.

With hysteresis the interval following a sensed event may be _____ than the LRI.

Rate hysteresis does not occur after a _____ event.

LONGER
PACED

CASE 34 (✳✳)

A 57-year-old female with a history of coronary artery bypass graft surgery and VVI pacemaker for sick sinus syndrome presents to the emergency room with crushing substernal chest discomfort of 2 hours duration. The patient is taken emergently to the cardiac catheterization lab. An ECG during ventricular pacing is obtained prior to catheterization.

Is there anything on it suggestive of acute myocardial infarction?

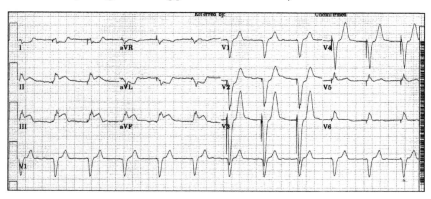

YES

There is ST depression in multiple leads where the QRS is predominantly negative, and there is ST segment elevation in multiple leads where the QRS is predominantly positive. These findings are all suggestive of acute myocardial infarction during ventricular pacing.

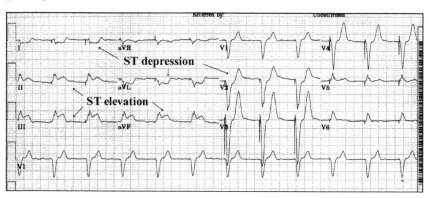

During cardiac catheterization she was found to have what appeared to be an acute thrombus of the bypass graft supplying the right coronary artery.

Ventricular pacing can mask the typical ST segment findings for acute myocardial infarction that one might see on a non-paced ECG. Had this been the case for this patient the treatment may likely have been the same given the patient's signs and symptoms suggesting acute myocardial infarction.

Findings on a ventricular paced ECG that are suggestive of acute myocardial infarction include ST segment elevation in leads where the QRS is predominantly _____, ST segment elevation ≥5 mm in leads where the QRS is predominantly _____ and ST segment _____ in leads where the QRS is predominantly negative.

POSITIVE, NEGATIVE, DEPRESSION

Case 35 (✱✱)

A 65-year-old male has a dual-chamber defibrillator implanted for ventricular tachycardia. The device is programmed with back-up bradycardia pacing, DDD 60/200/120 PVARP 200 ms. He has no known deficit in AV conduction. On the evening after implantation he develops the sudden onset of a rapid heartbeat. The resident seeing the patient obtains an ECG and treats the rhythm with medication for presumed AF.

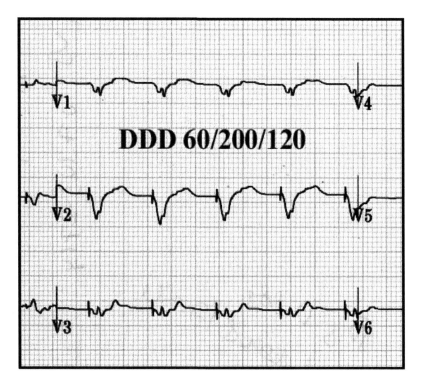

By the next morning the rapid rhythm has remained unchanged. You perform a single programming change and the rhythm returns to normal.

What happened?

PMT RESOLVED WITH INCREASED PVARP

The patient is paced in the ventricle at upper rate (120 bpm [500 ms]). There are also P waves buried in the T waves with each beat, each occurring after the PVARP. This is consistent with PMT.

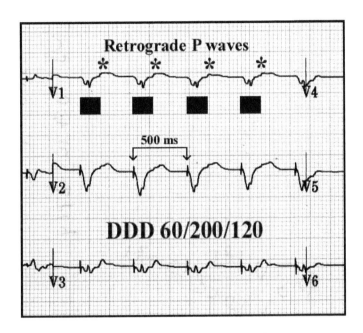

Increasing the PVARP caused each retrograde P wave to not be sensed, thus returning the rhythm to normal. Why wasn't a magnet placed on the device to temporarily break the rhythm first? Placement of a magnet on a defibrillator has the potential for *turning off* the delivery of tachyarrhythmia treatments! Thus, placement of a magnet over a defibrillator should only be undertaken by individuals experienced with their use on defibrillators.

Management Solution: Follow for adequate PVARP to prevent PMT.

Delivery of tachyarrhythmia functions of an implanted defibrillator may be _____ _____ by placing a _____ over it.

TURNED OFF, MAGNET

CASE 36 (✷✷✷✷✷)

You are called by your office regarding a 53-year-old female with a dual-chamber pacemaker previously implanted by another physician for CHB and paroxysmal AF. She is undergoing a stress test. Initially an AV sequentially paced rhythm is noted, however during the recovery phase the rhythm changes. A nurse is concerned that there may be a "pacemaker problem."

Is there a problem, and if so, what is it?

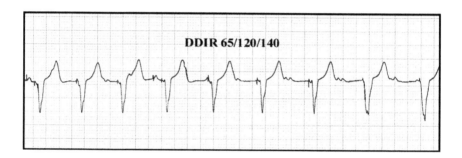

NORMAL DDIR FUNCTION DURING ATRIAL TACHYCARDIA WITH CHB

The atrial rhythm became atrial tachycardia. The atrial waves sensed outside of the refractory periods inhibited atrial pacing. Because they did not conduct down the native conduction system, AV synchrony was lost with these beats and ventricular pacing at the sensor indicated rate ensued. The sensor indicated interval increased from 650 ms to 870 ms by the end of the strip. Only during the first and fourth beats was AV synchrony maintained, as no atrial sensing occurred. This resulted in AV sequential pacing at the sensor indicated rate.

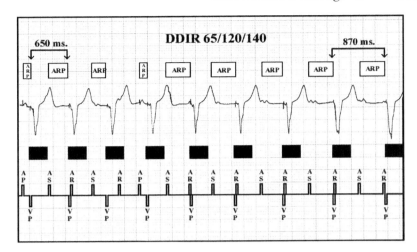

Management Solution: Reprogram mode to DDDR with mode switching on so as to: 1) not track rapid atrial rhythms and 2) maintain AV synchrony even in the face of CHB when rapid atrial rhythms are not occurring.

In the DDI(R) mode AV synchrony may not be maintained with CHB during periods of atrial _____.

SENSING

Case 37 (❋❋)

An 18-year-old male with a pacemaker implanted for neurocardi-ogenic syncope has the following ECG rhythm strip.

What can be said about the integrity of pacing and sensing function?

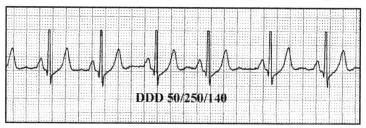

VENTRICULAR PACING → UNKNOWN
ATRIAL PACING → UNKNOWN
VENTRICULAR SENSING → INTACT
ATRIAL SENSING → UNKNOWN

There is no pacing seen so the integrity of pacing function is not known from the rhythm strip alone. Also, the state of atrial sensing is unknown because the PR interval is less than the AV interval and the VA interval is less than the R-R interval (the rhythm strip would look the same, complete pacing inhibition, whether atrial sensing was or was not intact). In each of these instances, though, ventricular sensing must be intact!

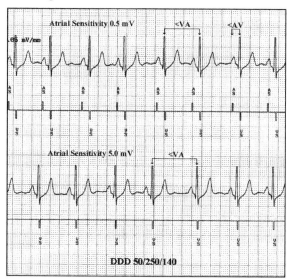

Management Solution: Utilize the pacemaker programmer to assess pacing and sensing function by temporarily altering pacemaker programming.

The integrity of atrial and/or ventricular pacing and sensing functions may be evaluated by utilizing the pacemaker _____.

The integrity of atrial sensing _____ be determined from a rhythm strip displaying no pacing when the PR interval is greater than the AV interval.

PROGRAMMER
CAN

Case 38 (✸✸✸✸✸✸)

A 46-year-old male with cardiomyopathy, severe first-degree AV block (400 ms PR interval), and a bi-ventricular implantable defibrillator presents to the emergency room with shortness of breath. A chest X-ray shows findings consistent with congestive heart failure (CHF) and all three pacemaker leads in the same position from that seen at implantation. An ECG is obtained of which the lead V_1 rhythm strip is shown below.

Is there anything on the strip that may explain the CHF?

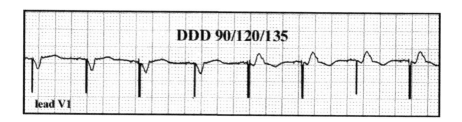

LOSS OF RIGHT VENTRICULAR (RV) CAPTURE

There appears to be AV sequential capture throughout, however the QRS complex changes to a wide (180 ms) RBBB morphology midway through the rhythm strip. This is indicative of loss of RV capture!

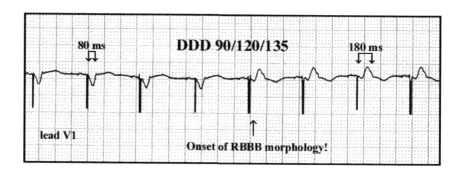

Pacing thresholds were obtained and revealed that the threshold of the RV pacing lead was elevated to the programmed output. Why do these QRS complexes not represent fusion versus capture beats? This patient had severe first-degree AV block, so no native conduction from the paced atrial complexes would have occurred prior to ventricular pacing.

Bi-ventricular pacing may improve cardiac performance in certain patients with CHF by resynchronizing electrical activation of both ventricles with respect to atrial activation. This may also result in a narrowing of the bi-ventricular paced QRS complex as compared to that without pacing. In the above example loss of RV pacing caused an increase of the QRS complex width to 180 ms when only left ventricular (LV) pacing was intact in the ventricles. This loss of ventricular resynchronization over time may have precipitated a worsened cardiac performance, and thus the CHF.

Management Solution: Increase ventricular pacing output to obtain reliable bi-ventricular capture.

Bi-ventricular pacing may improve cardiac _____ in patients with CHF.

PERFORMANCE

CASE 39 (✳✳)

A 64-year-old female with history of CHB and dual-chamber pacemaker is undergoing a treadmill stress test and suddenly complains of a "jump" in her chest during the study. The PVARP is 400 ms. The following ECG occurred at the time of onset of her symptoms.

What happened?

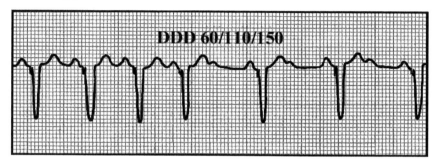

NORMAL MOBITZ TYPE II UPPER RATE BEHAVIOR

Her sinus rate increased until every other P wave began falling into the PVARP. This is Mobitz type II upper rate behavior. There was no change in the interval between sensed P wave and ventricular pacing spike prior to block because upper rate was not being infringed upon (total atrial refractory period [TARP] > URI). Had the TARP been less than the URI then Mobitz type I (prolongation of the AV interval prior to block) upper rate behavior would have occurred.

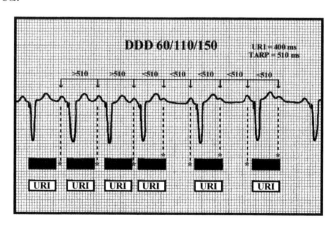

Some pacemakers have a function that can prevent such sudden changes in ventricular pacing during high P wave rates. They prevent this by pacing the atrium when it is determined that a significant interval has passed after a ventricular pacing output without sensing a P wave (i.e., as would happen when a P wave falls into the PVARP during upper rate behavior). This type of function is sometimes referred to as "rate smoothing."

Management Solution: Reprogram the URL higher (URI shorter) and PVARP shorter to prevent block, or if available, consider programming on a "rate smoothing" function.

Mobitz type II upper rate behavior can occur during P wave tracking when the TARP is _____ _____ URI, and Mobitz type I upper rate behavior can occur during P wave tracking when the TARP is _____ _____ URI.

GREATER THAN, LESS THAN

CASE 40 (❋❋)

A 73-year-old female with a dual-chamber pacemaker is admitted with heart failure. While undergoing telemetric monitoring her nurse notices the following rhythm and calls you concerned that the pacemaker is intermittently not working properly.

Are they right?

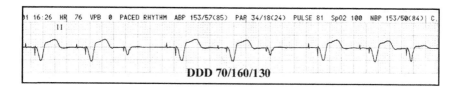

NORMAL FUNCTION WITH VENTRICULAR FUSION BEATS

Every third beat there is a premature atrial beat that is sensed. Measuring the AV interval backwards from the following ventricular pacing spike reveals the point of atrial sensing that initiated the interval. This occurs late in the P wave (i.e., after the atrium has been generously activated). By the time the AV interval has timed out in these instances native AV conduction has occurred, resulting in the ventricular fusion beats. There is no ventricular fusion after the atrial paced beats because the AV interval begins before the atrium has really been activated and times out before any native AV conduction can occur.

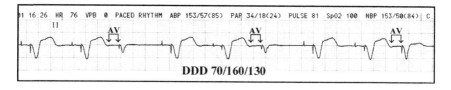

Pacemakers now have the ability to program two different AV intervals, one each depending on whether the atrium is sensed or paced. Since the AV interval starts before the atrium has really been activated with atrial pacing the AV interval is typically programmed longer. Conversely since the AV interval starts after the atrium has begun to be activated with atrial sensing the AV interval here is typically shorter. The result of having these two different AV intervals is a consistent timing of the ventricular hemodynamic event with respect to atrial contraction from both native and paced activation.

Management Solution: Program separate AV intervals for both atrial paced and sensed events.

In a pacemaker with separate AV intervals for atrial sensing and pacing, the AV interval is typically _____ following sensing than that following pacing.

SHORTER

CASE 41 (✻✻✻)

You are reviewing ECGs from the pacemaker clinic and come across this recording during AV sequential pacing.

Is there any reason to be concerned, and if so, why?

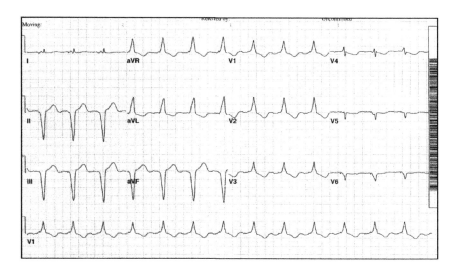

YES, RBBB VENTRICULAR CAPTURE MORPHOLOGY

Each ventricular beat shows an RBBB morphology!

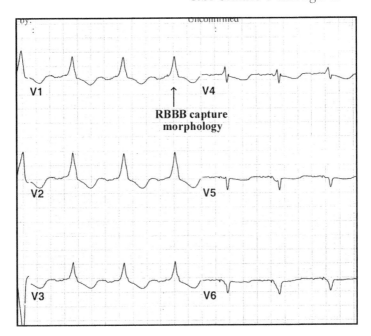

An RBBB capture morphology can be significant if the ventricular lead was originally placed via the transvenous route into the right ventricle. It indicates that the lead may have advanced into the left ventricle, and thus poses a potential risk for thrombus formation and stroke! In this case the ventricular lead was placed on the surface of the LV during an open heart surgical procedure and is no cause for concern.

Management Solution: None, unless only a RV lead was originally placed via a transvenous route. Withdrawal of the lead if confirmed to have advanced to the LV would then be needed.

An _____ ventricular capture morphology can occur with either a _____ ventricular lead that has advanced into the LV or an epicardial lead placed on the surface of the LV during _____ _____ _____.

RBBB, TRANSVENOUS, OPEN HEART SURGERY

CASE 42 (✸✸)

A 75-year-old female undergoes bypass graft surgery and has the following rhythm strip with pacing from a temporary external pacemaker (newer model) on the fourth postoperative day. After analyzing the rhythm you determine there to be a problem.

What is it?

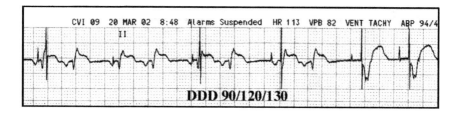

LOSS OF ATRIAL SENSING AND CAPTURE

Initially, there are atrial pacing spikes clearly occurring after P waves. Also there are ventricular pacing spikes occurring at a shortened AV interval following two of them (safety pacing!). This indicates loss of atrial sensing. It is likely that all other P waves are not sensed and the subsequent R waves inhibited both atrial and ventricular pacing in those cycles. At the end of the strip atrial pacing without capture appears to occur.

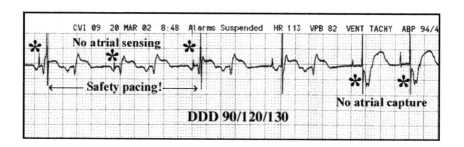

Temporary epicardial pacing wires are utilized in bypass graft and heart valve surgery patients as some patients may develop conduction system problems as a result of the surgery. Frequently the conduction disturbance may recover, however in some a permanent pacemaker is required. It is not unusual for the temporary pacing wires utilized in bypass surgery patients to malfunction, sometimes fairly early in the postoperative period.

Also, recall that the older models of temporary external pacemakers do not have safety pacing function, however newer models may as in the one used for this patient.

Temporary epicardial pacing wires may _____ in the post-surgery period.

Safety pacing is frequently an indicator of loss of _____ _____.

MALFUNCTION
ATRIAL SENSING

Case 43 (✳✳✳✳✳✳)

A 60-year-old male with an ICD implanted 2 days prior for ischemic cardiomyopathy and ventricular tachycardia presents to the emergency room after having received more shocks than he can count, all without warning. The physician implanting the device also inserted a pacemaker lead into a LV branch of the coronary sinus vein so as to provide bi-ventricular pacing given a history of significant CHF symptoms and left bundle branch block. Bi-ventricular pacing was accomplished by "Y-adapting" the right and LV leads (inserting both ventricular lead plugs into a special device that connects the leads together, thus allowing insertion into the single ventricular pacing/sensing port of the ICD). From the device, you obtain the following rhythm ECG and EGM sequence leading to one of the shocks.

What happened and what was the likely cause of the problem? The pacing mode is DDD 60/120/150.

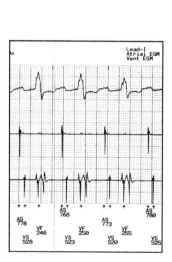
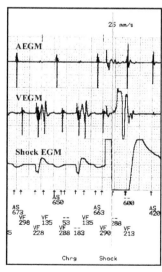

DISLODGMENT OF THE LV PACING LEAD BACK TO THE MAIN CORONARY SINUS, WITH RESULTANT LEFT ATRIAL SIGNAL ON THE VENTRICULAR EGM INTERPRETED AS A VENTRICULAR EVENT

There is a very large near-field component of the ventricular EGM that times out with late atrial activation on the surface rhythm strip, and is interpreted by the ICD as a sensed ventricular event (VS) with each beat. This occurs because the LV lead probably dislodged back to the main coronary sinus (recall that the coronary sinus lies in a groove between the left atrium and ventricle) and records a left atrial signal with each sinus beat. Because this lead is "Y-adapted" to the RV lead and plugged into the ventricular lead pacing/sensing port of the ICD, the ICD does not know any better than to interpret this large component as a ventricular event. Rate criterion for shocking was then met each time the sinus rate rose to a sufficient level (Ouch!). Chest fluoroscopy confirmed the diagnosis.

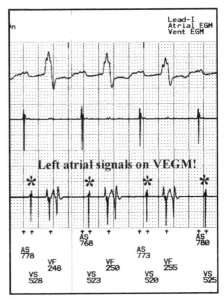

Also, note the absence of any ventricular signal recorded by the ICD's shocking coil at the time these events occur on the ventricular EGM. The ICD shocking coil in the right ventricle is not connected in any fashion to the LV lead.

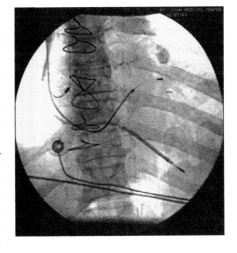

"Y-adapting" a LV coronary sinus lead to a RV lead and then inserting into a single ventricular pacing/sensing lead port can potentially put the patient at risk for adverse events when the lead dislodges back, such as described above. Another possible adverse event when the Y-adapted coronary sinus lead dislodges back to the atrium is when a patient has CHB and no native ventricular escape. The left atrial component recorded by the LV lead can be sensed and inhibit ventricular pacing with each cycle. This can be deadly!!

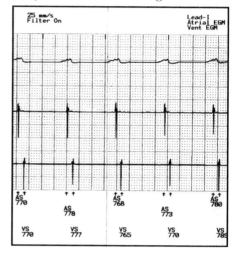

Management Solution: Until definitive inpatient management of the dislodged lead is undertaken, be it another attempt at repositioning in the LV venous anatomy (still at danger for dislodging again!) versus removal from the system: 1) turn off all tachycardia therapies, 2) reprogram the pacing mode to DDD with a very short AV interval. With the AV interval appropriately shortened the ICD will pace the right ventricle before the left atrial signal can be sensed by the LV lead to inhibit ventricular pacing. This will avoid complete ventricular pacing inhibition in the setting of CHB.

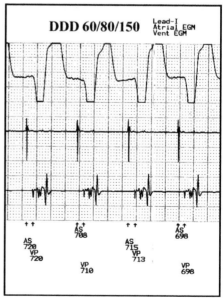

"Y-adapting" a left and RV lead together is potentially _____ when the LV lead dislodges backwards.

DEADLY

Index

Printed and bound by CPI Group (UK) Ltd, Croydon, CR0 4YY

Printed and bound by CPI Group (UK) Ltd, Croydon, CR0 4YY

27/10/2024

14580192-0001

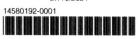